Ideas in Medicine™

by

Graeme Smith

web site; www.ideasinmedicine.com and

Twitter; @ideasinmedicine

Table of Contents

Introduction

This book scratches the surface of the medical/pharma industry - one of the biggest global industries.

I have attempted to show my personal experience in this amazing sector which has been very good to me and my family. I humbly admit to being a relatively small fry compared to others in the industry who have made a much larger impact. Nevertheless, my story shows you how, with a little effort and preparation, you can look to take your Idea in Medicine from the Eureka moment to commercialisation.

I had little initial desire to write this, and certainly did not think   I could possibly find the time. The story is changing all the time and future editions may have to update some of the projects.

Dedication

For the additional workload of writing this book, I have to thank Matt Kinsella. As I was preparing my Web site, www.ideasinmedicine.com, I called Matt to help with the social media campaign; and as I spoke through my needs, he said to me 'You know Graeme, you really should write a book! People will be interested to hear about your experiences.' It has been an interesting thing to do, and I thank Matt for encouraging me to do it. I also need to thank Matt for introducing me to Catherine Nix who works for Matt. Catherine is an ex Theatre (OR) Nurse now working in social media, and she has helped me edit and fine tune the content with a keen awareness of the medical environment. You can find Matt and Catherine on www.mattkinsella.com

My wife is also a Catherine and she has helped me to check grammar and flow. Ramsay McLellan, a close friend, has been a great help in reminding me of certain past experiences for the book, and has encouraged me to remove some paragraphs that may have got me into trouble.

My wife Catherine, in addition to putting up with me for nearly thirty years, is also a director in the main company, and handles all the things which need administrative attention to detail: banking, accounts, logistics, etc. She is my foundation. My rock. A psychology graduate from Dundee University, she has been an amazing wife and mother. We have two incredible children in Emma and Christopher. They are as different as chalk and cheese. They have experienced all our tough times as well as the good and sometimes great times. We have travelled the world together, and if nothing else, they both know it's a bigger world out there than just bonnie Scotland. In fact, as I write this, Christopher has been living in Iceland for over a year and working for Kerecis Ltd. Meanwhile, my daughter Emma is turning me into 'Grandpa G' in February 2016 when I am only 56! Too young to be a grandpa in my humble opinion. I still feel like a 20-year-old (with 36 years' experience) but I am SO looking forward to it. My Mum, Dad and Sister as well as Catherine's Mum and Dad have all contributed massively to our family experience through good times and bad and I am truly grateful to them for that.

As well as an amazing family I have worked with numerous people, many of whom are mentioned in the book. Some are only fleetingly mentioned and some not at all. I have had to decide which relationships are relevant to the story.

If you are not mentioned, please forgive me. If you are mentioned but only fleetingly, then please get back in touch as some great things are happening! What is clear is that so many of my true friends are there again and again - and continue to be there. As I wrote the book, it was amazing to see the thread of connections. Loyalty and friendship are two attributes that are difficult to put a value on. All I know is that those attributes work for me. It is also good for me to recognise how few friendships have fallen by the wayside, and the very few that have fallen were perhaps not true friendships in the first place.

My business is all about innovations, contacts and experience. Do not hesitate to get in touch if you think I can help. The story is far from finished and is a work in progress. Watch this space.

Eureka, Euphoria, Reality and Riches

The book has been written to help explain why so many of the Medical Industry's innovations come from the relationship between medicine and industry.

The people involved come from within those huge brain pools of medical professionals and commercial dynamos. Many of the amazing trends in medicine have come about after a Doctor somewhere in the middle of an operation or treatment thinks "this would be so much easier if I had a device that did "this" or "that".

Some Doctors have the time and energy to bring their Eureka ideas to the market. Many do not, and don't have the energy or any idea – or inclination – of where to start the process. They don't know how to protect their ideas, start the initial investigations into efficacy, build prototypes, licence for commercial use, do the necessary clinical studies, form a company, open their bank account, employ the people to do the basic work, fund the project, manufacture the product and then commercialise and get their idea out to other medical professionals on a commercial basis.

Some have done it and gone on to make a fortune, many have tried and failed. Often, their ideas get sucked into massive global commercial organisations and never see the light of day. That is what this book is all about. I want to help you bring your **Ideas in Medicine** to a commercial reality. Learning a little about me will help you build a picture of what makes me tick and explain some of my pathways.

I can only scratch the surface of the enormous world of medicine, and what you read about in these chapters will be my experiences in that world. The book is intended to shout out "**YOU** can bring your Eureka moment to reality".

Ideas in Medicine

The whole concept of **Ideas in Medicine** came about during the time LMA licenced their Urology business and the Stonebreaker device to Cook Medical in 2009. You'll read more about this later, but LMA or the Laryngeal Mask Airway Company had been recently acquired by Teleflex, and like many ideas that are turned into businesses, it came from spotting an unmet need. Invented by an anaesthetist who wanted an easier way to put patients to sleep before an operation. —"LMA" became a success story that grew into a company turning over multi millions. Importantly, they changed the way patients were handled pre and post op. They wanted to diversify and launched a Urology Lithotripsy device and I was called in to help their sales grow and expand internationally.

During this time, I started to reflect on how many ideas in medicine became realities. The name came in a moment of inspiration. As the idea came to me, I knew it was perfect. I ensured the domain name was available and at that time did not register the company but have done so since.

From day one I was clear about what Ideas in Medicine should be all about. I wanted to help medical people

11

around the world follow a definite supportive pathway to commercialise their ideas. The guidelines below are part of an initial guidance document I prepared.

Establish Your Business
First step in the process of commercialising your idea is the need to set up a business.

General guidelines will be offered from www.ideasinmedicine.com on the different business platforms you can choose to establish in this first step. Once you have established your business, you will need a bank account, to establish a relationship with an accountant, perhaps you will want a website, etc. The process can seem complex and daunting if you don't have a business background. However, you will find our support invaluable in the process.

Product Patent
The intricacies and ever-changing dynamics of patent law in emerging medical devices markets will be discussed at length on the Ideas in Medicine site. As device markets become more complex and more innovations are produced, legislative and regulatory systems need to adapt to the changing marketplace in order to preserve and protect one of the most valued commodities for medical device manufacturers: intellectual property.

Nevertheless, the adequate protection of intellectual property is critical for the sustained viability of the medical device industry, especially in emerging markets. Device manufacturers have to contend with patent law and intellectual property protection in a developing market; such as China, India etc. There are also ongoing concerns about potential changes to patent law in already established markets, including the EU and the US. www.ideasinmedicine.com will help guide you through these processes.

Regulatory Approval

The diversity of rules and regulations globally needs to be traversed with knowledge and professionalism. Guidance will be given on the needs for your idea and product approval - dependent on the markets being aimed at. The classification of your device will also determine the approach you need to develop. Regulatory approvals and protection of patents often proceed with a clear end point in mind – especially with the in depth specialist knowledge, protection and guidance.

Funding

One of the important decisions you will make early on is how you will fund your Idea. This can be self-funded of course, and your control can be fully retained. The cost of progress can surprise many people though. The costs can quickly escalate into hundreds of thousands. How you obtain your funding is also a key decision.

Do you go to a bank? A Business Angel? A Venture Capital firm? There are many companies out there with war chests of money looking for the next great **Idea in Medicine.**

I am sure many of us have been entertained watching Dragons Den on TV where a successful panel of entrepreneurs review ideas and decide whether to invest. Often, a big percentage of your company has to be handed over in exchange for the money. The key point here is that you often notice that the panel usually invest in business sectors they are familiar with. This is important as they fully appreciate that you are not just taking their money, but often, the key element is the investor's contacts, experience, support and knowledge. Those points are invaluable and should be part of your decision on who you decide to accept your funding from. The key thing about being part of the **Ideas in Medicine** network is that you will be able to seek support and clarity from our experts before you sign on any dotted line!

Manufacturing

Following the successful initial work on patent protection, regulatory approvals and product licensing, you will need to decide where to manufacture your product. Decisions such as these will be pivotal in the overall success and potential profitability of your idea. The global reach of www.ideasinmedicine.com will ensure you select your manufacturing base wisely, and with full knowledge of what support is available in each country. Certain countries in the world have built an excellent reputation for manufacturing medical devices whilst others are key centres in the manufacture of pharmaceuticals. Due to the impact on each country's economy of having a successful and growing manufacturing base in the medical industry, grants and incentives can often be obtained. The website will inform you of such opportunities.

Sales and Marketing

In many ways, sales is the most important part of the process. Some of the best ideas in the world have failed to make an impact because they have not been sold properly. We will have a global network of medical distributors for you to select from. These are specialised companies which have experience in your field, a fully trained sales force with contacts and key opinion leaders ready to discuss your medical product with.

Using a distributor network is the most cost effective way to reach the global medical market. Like all routes, there are strengths and weaknesses to each route to market. I often hear how a badly chosen distributor can be like a blockage in an artery as far as sales is concerned. They have many other products in their bag to sell. Yours will be just one of them. There are a number of good ways to ensure you get the attention of your distributors.

In some cases however, it may be that your investors advise a direct sales force fully controlled by your company. More expensive, BUT more control and focus. This route and that of a distributor network option will be fully discussed and debated with the **team at www.ideasinmedicine.com**

Medtronic

Every story has to have some references. This book has a clear storyline of medical ideas being nurtured into successful companies. I could never have guessed when I started how one particular company would feature so often. I have never worked for the company directly, but they have acquired companies I did work for, and amazingly, one of the most important companies in the middle of me writing this book. The company started from an idea in a garage - and now are turning over billions of dollars annually.

Medtronic was founded in 1949 in northeast Minneapolis by Earl Bakken and his brother-in-law Palmer Hermundslie as a medical equipment repair shop.

Through their repair business, Bakken came to know Dr. C. Walton Lillehei, a doctor in the field of heart surgery. Dr Lillehei was then at the University of Minnesota Medical School. They got talking about heart surgery, and in particular, heart pacemakers.

The deficiencies of existing pacemakers were made painfully obvious following a power cut over Halloween in 1957 which affected large sections of Minnesota and western Wisconsin. As a direct result of this electric blackout, a patient of Dr Lillehei's died. The child, who was a pacemaker dependent patient of Dr Lillehei died because the pacemakers in those days all needed a constant supply of electricity. The next day, Dr Lillehei spoke with Bakken about developing some form of battery-powered pacemaker. Stemming from this need, Bakken modified a design to create the first battery-powered external artificial pacemaker.

Bakken built a small transistor pacemaker that could be strapped to the body and powered by batteries. Work into this new product continued, producing an implantable pacemaker in 1960.

Medtronic grew into a multi-billion-dollar business from a few guys in a garage – and a clinician with a need and some good ideas. More about this later.

That's what this book is all about – **Ideas in Medicine**.

In June 2014, Medtronic announced its acquisition of Covidien, PLC of Ireland for $42.9 billion in cash and stock. This was the largest acquisition in its history (story to come).

The Covidien story, after it morphed from Tyco Healthcare's acquisition of United States Surgical Corporation is very much part of my story.

Medtronic is a global leader in medical technology – "alleviating pain, restoring health, and extending life for millions of people around the world" – is their company creed.

Quite a statement from Medtronic. I was not intending going into any details about my background but was advised my story will interest people. Especially my own personal early experiences in hospitals. So the next few chapters can be skipped if you are only interested in the Medical part.

Country Boy

I was born in a tiny village hospital in Scotland. It was in a place called Fyvie, a little village of about 1000 people. My Mum, Betty, was from Oldmeldrum and my Dad, Larry, was from Inverurie. Two equally tiny villages in the North East of Scotland. They were hard working Scottish parents and I enjoyed a loving supportive environment in which to grow up.

My amazing sister Gill was 2 years younger than me and we were brought up in Aberdeen in a council house with 2 bedrooms. Gill and I shared a room, and until I was about 10, that's how it was. Then, my Dad built a partition in the front bedroom and we each had our own small space. My parents still live in the same house in Mastrick, which is a council scheme on the outskirts of the city.

The school we went to, Summerhill Academy, was a notorious trouble spot. So bad the BBC made a 30-minute documentary about the school and its reputation for violence in and around the school. The BBC reckoned it was because of the clash of styles between two camps of teachers. Mr Mackenzie, the headmaster, was a liberal new style teacher, and his ideas were to bring the troublemakers in for "a chat" rather than the leather belt on the hands, while the other half of the teaching fraternity resorted to corporal punishment in order to control us.

I remember once heading into a technical department metal work lesson and some pushing occurred at the front door. The teacher lined us up - both boys and girls - and commanded us to raise both hands and he took the double-pronged, thick, leather belt off his shoulder. He proceeded to go along the line and belted us on each hand, and then when he reached the end of the line he went back again. We were about 12 years old. Sore, but the hardest bit was making sure nobody else saw it hurt, or you would become the next victim and butt of the jokes. Showing weakness was not advised at Summerhill Academy. Also, not very fair as most of the class were not doing any pushing but got punished anyway. Injustice lessons early on.

There was an unofficial league table amongst the guys, about who could get the most belt strokes in a year. A kind of rogues' gallery pride thing. It was scary getting from class to class as certain corridors were notorious ambush spots for the unwary. The school has now been knocked down, but there are, no doubt, many other similar stories of schools around the estates of the UK in the past.

Council House to School in a Bentley.

So school was tough and not a good environment to learn. Exam results were generally not good at Summerhill Academy. It was not a high-achieving school environment. However, as I look back now, I got an early break – literally. The work ethic in my family was always there, and from the age of 12, I delivered newspapers around the housing scheme. My Dad had left the army, having spent a lot of time in the Far East. The Argyle and Sutherland Highlanders were shipped to Korea towards the end of the war there. When my Dad got home and his national service was up, he got a job with the town council as a painter and decorator. This was his job until he retired. The job was not well paying, and my Dad would often work on "homers" at night and at the weekends where he could make some extra money. I would go with him occasionally, but it was boring and I didn't like it much. I now have an aversion to painting and the smell of white spirit. From an early age though, the work ethic was imprinted.

My Mum had various jobs, mainly part-time, and the one I remember was when she was a merchandiser for Jacobs Biscuits and she would go from supermarket to supermarket stocking up the shelves. She also worked in a meat factory called Lawson's of Dyce, and I remember how late she would get home at nights. It was a cold miserable environment to work in, but my Mum did it for years. Mum always wanted better for us and pushed us on to achieve.

Even though the money was always tight looking back, my sister and me had an amazing upbringing and we never wanted for anything. Mum and Dad always seemed to get us the things we wanted. We were always encouraged to try things and push ourselves. We had a good family environment.

I remember going to the local bicycle shop and Dad bought me a bright yellow Puch-branded racing bike. I loved that bike and spent hours cleaning it, making sure the brakes were right and lubricating and repairing burst tyres.

Anyway, on my paper round one dark winter's night cycling down Sheddocksley Drive, I was gawping at the light on the tarmac created by my brand new front cycle light, which I had got for Christmas. Next minute I had tumbled head over heels and had crashed onto the road. I had clipped a parked car with my left knee. I lay there for a while, luckily no cars were coming the other way, and knew something was up with my leg. I used the bike as a support and hobbled home sobbing.

Mum and Dad took me to the Emergency Department at the City Hospital. It was my bad fortune that the hospital was full of football fans being treated for stab wounds, concussions and various other injuries caused by a lot of trouble in the City, when the Glasgow teams came calling. Aberdeen fans were always "up" for a visit from the two Glasgow teams Celtic and Rangers. It was a part of the environment of football throughout Scotland at that time. That match is remembered as much for fan trouble inside the ground as out. One poor lassie had a knife stuck in her head which had been maliciously thrown from somewhere behind her in the stadium.

Suffice to say, it was chaos in the Emergency Rooms that night, and when my turn came for treatment, the staff completely missed the fracture in my tibia, which the X-ray should have shown up. So I was sent home. I knew something was not right though as I could feel the bones grinding together in my knee. Two days later I was back at the hospital. This time the fracture was spotted and I spent the next 6 months in a full-length plaster cast covering the whole foot, except my toes, all the way up to just below my groin. My first experience of morphine, but it wouldn't be my last.

It was very difficult to get around. In fact, an amazing teacher called Mr Sangster would come to my door and take me to school and helped my schooling from that point. He came to pick me up every morning in a classic old Bentley. Not many of those were seen in Mastrick. I remember the old leathery smell of the inside of the car.

I couldn't walk from class to class, and so they set up my lessons in the nurses' room and I would have my lessons taken down for me. No distractions, only time on my hands, boredom and with the odd visit from teachers and pupils. One welcome lass had a bit of a thing for me and some awkward fumbling would take place in that wee room. All the more exciting as the Admin staff were all in the rooms next door…. anyway I digress!

When the plaster came off something was not right. Apparently, the plaster had not been set right. I had a constant grinding pain, not in my knee where the tibia fracture had occurred, but in my ankle for some reason. It turned out that two bones had somehow fused together and the hospital gave me the great news for a 15-year-old at Summerhill Academy. I was going to have to wear a leg calliper for the rest of my life! Can you imagine! This leg calliper was a hideous contraption. Metal legs below the knee, and they had to be inserted by a joint into the heel of my daytime shoes permanently. It also made me limp. So from that point I was easy prey and separated from the herd. The mickey taking was pretty much constant.

I eventually cracked and one poor guy got it. In physics class, he was constantly calling me "cripple" and "peg leg" and the like and mimicking my limp. I said nothing. After class, I followed him out. I didn't wait for the playground or the home streets where most of the fights happened with everybody in a baying circle cheering on the participants. I went up to him, grabbed him by the hair and brought his nose down on my knee. As he fell, I set about him pretty bad until I was pulled off. I feel guilty about that to this day. I went home and said nothing to my folks until the teachers arrived at the door to tell them what had happened.

During the discussions that followed this incident, I said that the thought of the calliper and pain for the rest of my life was depressing me. The hospital kept saying there were no other options. Nothing they could do. Hospital and clinical incompetence is not surprising to me now, but back then, doctors seemed infallible. So the family took what they said as sacrosanct.

Mr Sangster had other ideas. We made an appointment and he pretended he was my Dad. He was pretty cultured and spoke with gravitas. He questioned the doctors during the appointment he arranged. Actually

26

more like grilled them. He dropped the word "incompetence" and "unprofessional" in a few times. Laid it on thick. After some time, guess what, there WAS something they could do. However, there was only one Consultant Orthopaedic surgeon who could do the operation, and he worked between Aberdeen and Dundee as he was very talented.

Pain for Gain

The hospital I was sent to after about 6 months of waiting was called Stracathro Hospital. It was an old World War 2 facility just off the main road between Dundee and Aberdeen. It was about 45 minutes' drive from Mastrick, so not easy to get to for my folks. Only my Dad had a driving licence and he was working, so I didn't get visitors every day. Not that it mattered, as I was so drugged up most of the time on morphine. I was hospitalised there for 2 weeks.

When I came around from the anaesthetic, I was in enormous pain from my ankle. I looked down and even the plaster cast was blood red, as the bleeding had not been stopped properly. I remember drifting in an out of consciousness for a few days. A few tears were shed when my folks arrived. Looking back, they dosed me up pretty good on the painkillers, and not just any painkillers, it was pretty much pure morphine I was given. Injected at first, and then tablet form. I got very used to the blanket-like warm glow from the drugs. Opiates often don't alleviate certain pain, but they make it that you don't seem to mind it. You tolerate the pain better.

When I eventually got back home, the pain was still there and the latest plaster cast was a feature for eight more

28

months, so it felt hopeless trying to alleviate the constant pain. I couldn't even touch my leg. The pain killers helped of course, but after quite a while, I can't remember how long now, they suddenly stopped giving me the pills. I crashed. It was like going 'cold turkey' from heroin. I remember the feelings now like it was yesterday. I was agitated, upset, emotional, sick and in pain. Not a nice time.

Eventually, after 8 months, the plaster cast came off. My left leg was weedy and thin as the muscles had wasted away. What was clear after a number of weeks though was that the pain had gone. No pain for the first time in a couple of years. Then started the physiotherapy to get me mobile again. To this day, I do not have mobility in my ankle. I can move it up and down but can't rotate it. However, I don't wear a calliper now and don't limp (much). I was pretty much given a new lease of life. Drugs though were a large part of my life during that period. Prescribed drugs. It was not long before I was dabbling in other drugs. They were readily available in Aberdeen because of the booming oil industry and the large number of Americans and Canadians brought in to service the jobs that local people had no skills to do initially.

Looking back, that leg break experience was a formative part of my early life. The thing is, during that leg injury period, I studied. Pretty much non-stop with no distractions, I studied. It meant I ended up with 8, O-levels and 4 Higher grades which gave sufficient qualifications to go to University or College. At that time in Aberdeen, the oil boom was kicking in and engineers were needed. So I was encouraged to apply for Robert Gordon Institute of Technology and the course was a BSc in Engineering.

Drop Out

I was music daft from an early age. Another thing my parents did for me was to pay for guitar lessons for me. I also took lessons at school and learned to play the classical guitar. I ended up with a grade 5 classical guitar qualification. I loved my guitar, and when they saw I was serious, they bought me a Tatra Classical guitar, which I still have to this day.

I played the guitar almost every day. Not a day went by when I didn't practise and play. I learned to read music. I stayed on at school for a fifth year and was accepted for Robert Gordon's Technical College (Now Robert Gordon's University).

I bought the New Musical Express every week and knew all about the upcoming bands and who was doing what. Pretty soon, the word got out that I could play a bit and my Mum's pal said her son played keyboard and he had a pal who played drums. So Ron Brown, Walt and I formed a band. We focussed on playing cover versions and eventually got a few gigs. We pottered about for a while as drummer, lead guitar and rhythm guitar. Then a guy called Marsh came along who could play bass. We were off. Then somehow between school and college, Marsh and I saw an ad in the local paper looking for summer workers in the Netherlands. A little village, called Ossterhaut, near Nijmegan. We were off to live in a village farm commune with about thirty other young British students. We worked in a pickle factory Monday to Friday in a boring factory packing gherkins into jars. The farmer was clever; we only got paid half our money and the other half was put into a bank account, which we got when the summer season was over. Weekends were great. Amsterdam was close and we would find our way into Amsterdam to buys drugs, alcohol and chase girls. It was a great summer and I came home on the ferry and had quite a bit of cash. I bought a Yamaha SG2000 guitar and a Burman amp – I had taken an acoustic guitar with me of course.

When I got back, I was approached by a more established "cooler" band and they asked me to join them. So I did. I liked the fact these guys were older, looked cool and always had drugs and girls around. This band had a van, a manager and even roadies and so off I went. Benny the lead singer and I were close. Dave Ross the bass Guitarist, Rob Wainright on the keyboards and Addi Addison on drums. A couple of variations to the line up over the years but those were the main guys. A lot of time was spent practising in cold empty halls, building up our repertoire of mainly covers but also a lot of our own songs.

Then, I started the BSc Engineering course at Robert Gordons Institute of Technology and lasted all of three weeks before I decided – nope – this is not for me! The frustrating part of being a drop out is that it doesn't have that option for your LinkedIn profile. LinkedIn keeps asking me to complete my profile which I can't. I suppose it looks good being there – but now you know the truth of it – I was only there for a few weeks.

Much to my folks' utter dismay and disappointment, I dropped out! They were gutted – especially my Mum who was always pushing us to be better and do more. I remember walking along Union Street after I left the office of the Dean who had to interview me (with Mum there). He had given stern advice about the path I was taking. I walked straight up to one of my favourite haunts, a trendy record shop called The Other Record Shop. Lots of cool people hung around here, and always the latest songs were being played. I asked for a job and they had seen me hanging around the shop for months. I was interviewed and offered a full-time job.

I thought all my Christmas's had come at once. I was made. Not only playing in a cool band, but working full-time in a cool record shop. This was a place where famous bands made promotional visits to promote records, sign autographs and meet people before their gigs.

Lunchtimes were very often liquid, and being the youngest of the staff members, I would just do what everybody else was doing. Drinking vodka and coke and then getting stoned on hash after lunch was the norm. People came in and bought records and we could play whatever we wanted on the sound system.

Meantime, our band was getting better and we built quite a following. We made recordings and bands like the Psychedelic Furs came to see us play at venues in Edinburgh. I spent quite a bit of time with them in Scotland and London. Drugs again were a big factor.

Our biggest claim to fame was we backed the Simple Minds during a concert in Aberdeen. Memorable because we got an encore, much to the lead singer Jim Kerr's annoyance as backing bands were not supposed to get encores. In fact, after the gig he burst into our dressing room and accused us of ripping off a guitar rift from one of their songs. Who knows, he may have been right. We were out of it most of the time.

It just goes to show what a small world it is though. My daughter Emma has recently gotten married, and Max my son-in-law's Dad is Mick MacNeil, who was the keyboard player in the Simple Minds. He remembers the gig way back when we were all just boys – because he was in a leg plaster. At a recent BBQ here at our house, he said "I remember you boys, you were good". I asked him to repeat what he said in front of my son Christopher, for a bit of street cred with my then 18-year-old lad Christopher who thought I was a complete divvy. The Simple Minds were a proper band and made it to the very top. We loved their music and style in those days. They were never the same after Mick left them.

So, band stuff at night, record shop during the day, rock star status just around the corner. All of that might have worked out if we had been a bit more focussed and were not spending more and more of our free time looking for our next drug high. We used to take loads of speed, either blues or amphetamine sulphate, which we used to either snort or inject. Heroin was always there, again often injected, and cocaine was available but usually too expensive for us. There was always more hash and oil around and not so much weed.

I was always ready. One working day, some dealers I knew came into The Other Record Shop. They had just turned over a fishing boat in the harbour and stolen the morphine from the first aid kit. Eejit here decided it would be a good idea to inject it and that's what I did. I remember to this day the rush hitting me like a warm bath from my head to my toes. I missed the feeling from my leg injury days. Then blackness.

I woke up 2 days later in a bed and I had no idea where I was. My colleagues had found me slumped in a heap in the staff lounge. They apparently panicked, not unsurprisingly, thinking I was just about to overdose and die. Not good for business. The Police always had their eye on the place as quite a few drug deals went down there. So, they somehow managed to get me to a flat around the corner where they put me on my side on the bed so I didn't choke on my vomit and kept an eye on me until I came around. What a waste that would have been, to have died of a drug overdose at age 22.

So the penny started to drop! What was I doing? Where was I going? Did I really want to live this life – what if I was less lucky next time? We had been living in a cottage outside Aberdeen. The place became notorious. It was always "open" for anybody looking to get wasted. The Police soon heard about it too and one morning, as were lying around, a dawn raid woke us up as the Police smashed in and started looking for the evidence. Someone had told them we were manufacturing amphetamines there! They quickly saw we were no danger to anybody (except ourselves) and had a chuckle when they went to our food cupboard and we had one raw turnip on the shelves for four lads. We didn't eat much in those days, other than carry outs, as the drugs suppressed our appetites.

That was the final straw, I quit drugs. Went cold turkey age 23. From age of 16 to 23 I had taken drugs in copious amounts every day, so coming off was not easy. I had experienced withdrawals before, after coming off the morphine following my leg injuries, so I knew what to expect. The physical symptoms were bad; sickness, lethargy, paranoia – but it was more the mental stuff. It had been such a large part of my life and all my friends were involved and they had no intention of stopping just because I wanted to. I went home to get cleaned up and get straightened up! My Mum was horrified when she saw the mess of my arms with the track marks (needle holes and bruises from the injections). Anyway, that was the start of my rehabilitation, and life getting back to some form of reality and normality.

Of course the band environment had not changed but I had. So, it was quickly obvious that the guys in the band and I were going in totally different directions. So I took the decision to leave the band. That didn't go down well either, but I knew there was too much temptation around, and I probably wasn't strong enough to resist it. So I left the band, left the cottage and went back home for a while. At age 23 with no job, no prospects and still a huge gap in my life where the band and drugs had been, I had to get busy.

From Druggie to Sales Rep

I was offered a part-time job as a student porter at the local hospital. Instead of being in a hospital as a patient, I was able to see the inner workings of a hospital. As well as normal dogsbody porter jobs; cleaning windows, sweeping floors, delivering goods and packages, we also had to wheel the patients to the Theatre (OR) AND with a great deal of trepidation, wheel dead patients to the hospital morgue. Anyway, it got me working and into a day-to-day routine.

While working, I knew this was not me, and I used to ask who the smart young "suits" were arriving in new cars. I was told those were the company reps. It never dawned on me how a company might be prepared to give somebody a car as part of their package. I liked that idea, and from that point thought to myself 'That's the job for me – how do I get into that game?'

One of the roadies for the band, who I kept in touch with, was working for a fruit machine company delivering machines to pubs and clubs around the Aberdeen area. He said his company was looking for a new sales rep. He didn't fancy it because you had to wear a suit and tie. So I went and got myself a cheap suit and borrowed a tie and applied for the job. Sometimes, in fact many times, life lends a hand. I went to that interview without a clue about what being a sales rep involved and had done no research into the company. I was seeing the Office Director Jack Talbot. Jack was in his sixties and had helped build Woolfson Leisure, one of the biggest suppliers of fruit machines, pool tables and juke boxes in Scotland.

I was in his office for ten minutes when he said "Right son, come with me". Next thing I know, I am in the front of his Mercedes and heading to Aberdeen fish market to help Jack pick up some fresh fish. He offered me the job and sent me home with my first company car. When I turned up at home, my Dad didn't believe it was my car to use. It was only a year old and why would anybody give me a car!? I was barely off the drugs and cleaned up! That's how I got my first full-time job and started my career in sales!

What a baptism that was. My job was to cold call pubs and clubs in the North East of Scotland, to convince them our machines were better than other companies in competition with Woolfson Leisure.

Can you imagine a young sprog walking in to some of the rough dockland pubs of Aberdeen asking "to see the proprietor", because that opening line was the extent of my sales training! It was a tough learning curve being the entertainment for drunken oil workers and fishermen! I learned fast, I had to.

In many ways, it was a great year because I didn't know any better and just got on with it. My results were good. I am sure I got more than a few "pity sales". Anyway, before long, as well as the famous PacMan video game, which I helped to sell, a new phenomenon hit the pub and club scene. Large screen TV and video recorders to show sports and films. This was cutting edge stuff back then.

I did well and we attended a licenced trade convention in Glasgow. The new manager of this division watched me work on the booth and basically offered me a job working for his division in Glasgow.

I liked the idea because it meant getting away from the temptations of Aberdeen, so I accepted. Within two weeks I was on my way to Glasgow and my first accommodation was in a bedsit in Great Western Road, and something amazingly strange happened. I walked into a pub in Byres Road Glasgow for a drink, and as I walked up to the bar, somebody shouted my name. I turned and saw one of the main drug dealers we used to buy our drug supplies from. I couldn't believe it! There he was in front of me asking "what are you doing here in Glasgow pal? I have some great gear back in the flat. Do you want sorting out?" That was my moment. My test.

Life changing. I can't remember exactly how it happened but I made some excuse and walked out the door. It was all a bit of a blur, but I remember thinking "WHAT!!!". I walked out, and to this day, I have never seen him again in or around Glasgow! After the bedsit, I moved to an even cheaper dump of a hotel called the Davenport Hotel, which has since been knocked down. It was all I could afford.

Again, a hard learning curve, but the job training was better and I was even sent to London for my first official Sales Training and Negotiation Skills course. I so loved that training course. I made it an enjoyable habit to constantly self-train and develop, and spent money regularly on Nightingale Conant training and motivational courses.

Without realising it, I nearly met my wife during one of the Big Screen installations. I was installing a system into the Student Union at Dundee University and Catherine was there, working in the bar to supplement her income, during her Psychology Degree course. She remembers the system being installed. Anyway, the meeting would come later.

So, there I was with a great job and had a great social life with my pal Stuart Robertson from my Tae Kwon Do class in Aberdeen (which I started during my clean up). In fact,

I went too far in my quest to clean up. I was almost a fanatic for martial art training, macrobiotic diets, mediation and exercise. Stuart was a trainee teacher in East Kilbride, and by then, I had bought a flat in the East side of Glasgow. We enjoyed our weekends drinking and chasing girls. We met some great neighbours in Glasgow too. Young East end Glasgow guys. Billy Butler was the first contact, and to this day – even though 30 years have passed – I see Stuart and Billy for a drink or two socially.

From Drug Rehab Volunteer to Husband

One day, sitting at home in the evening, I picked up the local paper and saw a story about a local initiative in Possil, Glasgow, one of the roughest housing schemes in the city. Possil has a notorious drug scene. The support idea was initiated by some local families and they had no funding or help from the Council. They basically worked with the local Priest. He had given up his big manse and The Place (that's what it ended up being called "The Place") was converted into 6 bedrooms where local youngsters could come, and in a supportive environment, clean up off the smack (heroin), which was so easy and cheap to get in the city. I thought I could help. It was mainly people volunteering who had little or no experience of the drug culture, other than what they saw it was doing to their children and society. So, 24 hours a day, 7 days a week, The Place was supported. I went along, was interviewed, was honest about my own past, and started volunteering.

I would attend a couple of hours on a Saturday or Sunday afternoon. The youngsters quickly realised that I had a good idea what was going on with them. Some were serious about cleaning up, some were not. I could speak their language and could tell quite quickly what their main motivation for being there was. I like to think we helped quite a few youngsters. Sadly, we would often see the same faces after a few months. I would sometimes take these youngsters out in my car into the country. In fact, to locations not far from where I live now. Many of these kids had not set foot outside the city very often – if at all.

Another life-changing event occurred after a couple of years helping out. One day, the Priest came in and said "Graeme this is Catherine, she is on your shift, look after her and show her the ropes". I was instantly attracted to her. What can I say, love at first sight? Well, the attraction was very strong from the start. I was determined to do the right thing from the start. I was already going out with a lass, but it was not going anywhere. So I ended that and didn't hedge my bets. I didn't want any of my dodgy past coming into this relationship. After a week or so, I asked Catherine out. She had been told about the Place looking for volunteers by her Dad. She had never taken drugs, and her Dad, John, was a Fire Officer in Glasgow. Catherine had wanted to do some volunteer work after graduating from Dundee University.

During dinner at an Italian Restaurant in Glasgow – our first date – she told me a funny story. When she had started the volunteer work, John and Lydia, her loving

Mum and Dad, were understandably nervous about their daughter working with reforming Junkies in Possil, Glasgow. Catherine tried to reassure them that she was being looked after by an ex-druggie (me) who was showing her the ropes. Can you imagine what they felt when they heard I had asked their daughter on a date! I didn't even get to meet them when I rolled up all nervous to their front door. She was out the door like a whippet and into the car with the front door quickly closed behind her.

We have been married 27 years now, and so hopefully, they have got over the shock. Her Dad, John, and Mum, Lydia, have been great in-laws. A terrific support for our family and always there if we need them!

In our married life, we have had many more ups than downs. We're a good match. Catherine is calm (most of the time), balanced and thoughtful, whereas I have always been a risk taker with high energy and can't sit still. I am sure many of the paths we have taken would not have happened if Catherine had not been such a faithful trustful partner. She never held me back from trying anything. Now, after 27 years, we look back and she laughs and has often said that life with me has never been boring!

I can see it now that without Catherine there, my own life

may easily have gone off the rails again. We are a good team and now Catherine is a director of our company and owns 50% of the shares. I would not have it any other way. I know there are many horror stories about marriage break ups and the fallout for assets afterwards. I wouldn't even blink in terms of a straight split – if it ever came to that - which I obviously hope it won't ever need to be thought about. It is only fair and Catherine has allowed me to drive on in terms of business creation where she looks after logistics, banking, accounts, human resources and administration. That suits Catherine fine as she has never been comfortable at the front end where I do my best work.

Also, what a great mother she has been. In the midst of our business ups and downs, we have had two wonderful children. My daughter Emma was born first. On the 23rd March 1991, after Catherine had endured a 24-hour labour, Emma was plonked into my lap as I sat in my hospital greens. The labour was long and then got complicated. The doctor came to see me and said Emma was in distress as the position she had settled in the womb was wrong and Catherine was going to have to be taken into Theatre (OR) for an intervention.

I was taken by the young doctor, who I now know was a Senior Registrar on the night shift, and shown how to get dressed into hospital greens and clogs. Who would have known that a few short years later, I would be showing others how to do the same and would be completely comfortable in theatre attire. When I look back, my association with hospitals has always been an important part of my life.

Emma came into the world and immediately became the centre of our focus. Now I really had to get my act together to provide not just for my wife – who was working full time as a careers officer back then – but our new arrival. The arrival of a child is a spectacular event, and we set about our parenting as best we could as all young couples do.

Four years later, Christopher arrived. Different scene altogether. Emma and I went round to her Granny and Papa's house and called the hospital. We were told nothing would happen until 5pm and we should come in then. Around 3pm the phone rang and Emma answered the phone (she was only 4 but very chatty already) and came through and said. "I have a little brother"!

We were all a little shocked and I was real disappointed, as I wanted to be there for the birth of my son. Anyway, the birth went well and Christopher literally popped into the world. He was healthy and the birth was smooth and uneventful – if not a little faster than everybody expected.

My son had two mothers from that point, with Emma taking on the role with great enthusiasm. Christopher was a beautiful baby boy with big eyes and bright nature. As time would go on, we found as well as generally having a lovely nature, he had his Mum's character trait of being a little volcano. When Catherine loses her temper – which doesn't happen very often – stand well back. It's explosive. Christopher was the same. The little guy had a temper that was just as explosive. So there we were, the Smith family.

Up the Ladder

After 5 years with Woolfson Leisure, a Recruitment Consultant called Tim Amatt approached me. He had a job for a vending salesman with General Foods, a blue chip company which sold Maxwell House coffee amongst many other brands. The job was selling coffee vending machines into business. The appeal was strong, and even though I was offered more money to stay with Woolfson Leisure, I decided the challenge of a blue chip environment appealed. I was immediately sent to Cheshire for a two-week training course and started my training.

Within the first quarter, I was Salesman of the Month and set about doing what I like to do – selling. The job at General Foods was a great experience and I learned a lot. It was always important for me that I kept learning and developing.

After I had proven myself in that environment, I got a surprise offer from the Recruitment Consultant who placed me in the job, offering me a position working with him. The appeal was instant and I learned the recruitment ropes. I loved being a Recruitment Consultant as I was still selling. Selling my service to clients. The added benefit was that to learn about the particular sales environment, I often had to shadow their sales teams. That allowed me to experience many diverse sales environments such as Canon, Gillette, Cussons, Boots Pharmaceuticals and various other companies. Totally invaluable! My recruitment skills were totally geared towards Sales and Sales management candidates. That was my growing expertise. I thrived on it. I also got involved in training. We used to train first line managers of different companies to recruit for themselves.

That role really taught me a ton about running a business, as I had to run myself as an Independent profit centre. I was responsible for my income and expenditure, profit and loss etc. It didn't start out that way, but moved to that model after some discussions with the owner Tim Amatt. It was a great learning curve on the realities of running a business as opposed to being an employee. I was now self-employed. In fact, when I think about it, almost from that point in 1990, I always considered myself as self-employed even though I was in employed positions after that. To my mind, it was always in the interests of the employer for me to think that way, as I was always looking to add value, not just collect a wage.

Even though I found myself in other employed positions in the future, I had the attitude that it was down to me to make things happen. I never looked on any position as a role I could coast through. It's always about delivery and building sales revenues for any product that's essential.

While working on recruitment projects, we spent a lot of time scanning the recruitment pages. It helped us to see who was doing what and the kind of roles up for grabs. It also gave us the chance to send candidates for selection.

One day, I spotted a small semi-classified ad of around 6 lines which intrigued me personally. It talked about a 6-week training course in the USA. That really got my attention. Very few companies invest so much time and money in developing new employees. I applied!

Following 5 interviews, a psychometric test and a visit to an operating theatre (Operating Room or OR) in the Sothern General Hospital Glasgow, I was told I was going to be sent to Norwalk, Connecticut for the training. I was delighted although nervous. I had never been away for the family for such a long time, but something told me I should do this.

Medical Device Sales On Steroids

I had no idea when I applied for the job with United States Surgical Corporation (Auto Suture Ltd in the UK) just how significant this company would be to my future.

The training course for the United States Surgical Corporation was as tough and challenging as it comes for any medical device company. In fact, the course was renowned for its high dropout rate. The pass level after 6 weeks of intense, 7 days a week, almost 18 hours a day full on activity was 95%. No pass – No job! The pressure was intense and was designed to ensure complete comprehensive knowledge of our products and our competitors' products.

We were trained to "wet scrub" which means to be at the operating table during the procedures while the operations were taking place. We were to give verbal technical assistance to the surgeons during live operations. We were taught to close sales at the operating table American style. Although I quickly worked out on returning to the UK that building relationships was a better and more productive way to obtain sales.

We trained in "wet labs" and were trained to suture,

staple, cut and use diathermy. There were daily role plays and assessments. Our evenings were spent studying together in this boot camp military style environment. The feeling of achievement when my results of 98.5% was announced remains with me to this day.

Then when we returned to the UK, we quickly found that scrub techniques were different and we had to adapt. The company farmed us out to company-friendly surgeons who continued to train us and we were "scrubbed up" every day, often at night, as the surgeons would use us as assistants – unpaid by them, of course!

Why did we do it? The environment we worked in was rarefied and felt privileged. We saw things many people never see. Also, the money and returns were good. Some of the sales guys were making seven figure commission sums which attracted some of the best sales professionals globally. Make no mistake, USSC or Auto Suture as it was known in the UK was a sales organisation and we were expected to deliver sales and hit our targets.

The training was generally regarded as the toughest in the Medical Device Industry and set standards. We effectively went through a crash course in surgery with training involving; Anatomy, Physiology, Surgical Terminology, Surgical Procedures, Aseptic Techniques, Surgical Stapling, Surgical Suturing, Sterilisation, Instrument

Applications, Competitive Products, Side-by-side comparisons, Role Plays, Theatre(OR) Protocol and various Laboratory Hands on Sessions.

It was after we got back we realised how important this training was. As I have said, it was our job to scrub up and provide "verbal technical assistance" during live procedures with patients on the table, but often, we did much, much more than provide verbal technical assistance. Our specific knowledge on the techniques about to be performed meant we were often called upon to conduct supportive tasks during the procedures. Often, hospitals were short-staffed, and we grew into valuable members of the operating room team.

It was always amazing to me, especially given my background, to find myself in that environment. I still do find myself in that environment these days, although my work now tends to be more international than in the UK.

United States Surgical Corporation (Auto Suture Ltd)

Surgical staplers were originally developed to address the perceived problem of patency (security against leaks of blood or bowel contents) in anastomoses in particular. Leaks from poor suturing of bowel anastomoses (join) was at that time a significant cause of post-surgical mortality. More recent studies have shown that with current suturing techniques, there is no significant difference in outcome between hand sutured and mechanical anastomoses, but mechanical anastomoses are significantly quicker to perform.

The technique was pioneered by a Hungarian surgeon, Humour Hultl, known as the "father of surgical stapling". Hultl's prototype stapler of 1908 weighed eight pounds (3.6 kg), and required two hours to assemble and load. Many hours were spent trying to achieve a consistent staple line and reliably patent (open) anastomoses.

The early instruments, by developers including Hultl, von Petz, Friedrich and Nakayama, were complex and cumbersome to use. The technology was refined in the 1950s in the Soviet Union, allowing for the first commercially produced re-usable stapling devices for creation of bowel and vascular anastomoses. Mark M. Ravitch, brought a sample of a stapling device after attending a surgical conference in USSR, and introduced it to entrepreneur Leon C. Hirsch, who founded the United States Surgical Corporation in 1964 to manufacture surgical staplers under its Auto Suture brand.

Until the late 1970s, USSC had the market essentially to itself, but in 1977 Johnson & Johnson's Ethicon brand entered the market and today, both are widely used, along with competitors from the Far East. Thus was born an amazingly acrimonious relationship between USSC and Ethicon. The lawyers made millions and millions of dollars handling the lawsuits regularly flying between both companies.

USSC was bought by Tyco Healthcare in 1998, which became Covidien on June 29, 2007. Tyco paid $3.3 Billion for U.S. Surgical! Talk about Ideas in Medicine paying off, but I have highlighted the story and history of stapling to show how long an "exit pay day" can sometimes take. Persistence and a vision are vital to it all. Since I started writing this book Medtronic have now acquired Covidien.

In the early days of surgical stapling, nobody gave it a chance. Why would anyone pay for a $300 stapler when the suture costs were $50 maximum? However, the safety and patency of mechanical (stapled) bowel anastomoses was being widely studied. It was generally the case in such studies that sutured anastomoses were either comparable or less prone to leakage. It is possible that this was the result of recent advances in suture technology, along with increasingly risk-conscious surgical practice. Certainly, modern synthetic sutures are more predictable and less prone to infection than catgut, silk and linen, which were the main suture materials used up to the 1990s. However, the company persisted and kept going.

One key advantage of surgical stapling was that it was much quicker. Another feature of the intestinal staplers is that the edges of the stapler act as a haemostat, compressing the edges of the wound and closing blood vessels during the stapling process.

Over the years, USSC aggressively kept growing. This was achieved by recruiting some of the best sales people from all over the world and paying them handsomely for success. Paying them very very well!!

As mentioned earlier, on May 26, 1998 Tyco International Ltd., an international manufacturing and service company on an acquisition spree, announced that it would acquire the United States Surgical Corporation for $3.3 billion in stock. Tyco is one of the world's largest makers of fire protection systems, a major provider of electronic security services and a leader in disposable medical products and underwater telecommunications systems.

The acquisition would help round out its line of medical products and help leverage its existing sales force by allowing it to sell more items to hospitals. U.S. Surgical's product lines include surgical staplers, sutures, electro-surgical products and disposable laparoscopic instruments. These products account for 90 percent of the company's revenues, which totalled $1.4 billion in 1997. By comparison, Tyco had revenues of about $13 billion.

Dennis Kozlowski (currently in prison in the USA for Corporate fraud), chairman and chief executive of Tyco said "With this transaction, Tyco will have $4.5 billion in medical product sales, a solid presence in the operating room and a greatly expanded array of products for use throughout the hospital." Tyco was based in Bermuda and had United States headquarters in Exeter, New Hampton. Under Mr. Kozlowski's leadership, Tyco's spending spree reached $10.5 billion in 1997.

Makers of medical products had been frequent targets of Tyco. In December 1997, it said it would buy the Sherwood Davis & Geck unit, a maker of needles, syringes and surgical sutures, for $1.77 billion in cash from the American Home Products Corporation. In April, it said it would acquire the closely held Confab, a maker of adult diapers and hygiene products.

United States Surgical Corporation had attracted takeover speculation for some time. It was without a clear heir apparent for Leon C. Hirsch, the chairman and chief executive, who was 70 years old back then. In the field of medical products where many companies were trading at vast multiples of earnings, several companies besides Tyco were said to be interested in U.S. Surgical, including Medtronic, Boston Scientific and Johnson & Johnson.

Anne P. Malone, an analyst at Salomon Smith Barney, said in a recent research report that her target price for U.S. Surgical stock was only $38 a share under the company's current leadership. "We do admit that a purchaser could look to a higher value," she wrote, "since there is the opportunity to recognize synergies." So, with the constant cash flow issues affecting US Surgical and the hated J&J circling, Leon Hirsch decided to sell.

Tyco, which had a market capitalization of $32 billion, said it expected the merger to lead to cost savings of $150 million over three years, with a third of the total coming from consolidation in manufacturing and distribution. Many companies were trading wildly above their values back in the heady pre-crash days.

Shares of Tyco, which was then a Wall Street darling, had risen 24 percent in 1997, while the stock of U.S. Surgical, viewed tepidly by analysts, had risen 34 percent because of all the takeover speculation. Mr. Hirsch was to remain head of U.S. Surgical, which was based in Norwalk, Connecticut. The company was to keep its name and be merged with other Tyco subsidiaries.

The other key person in the success of USSC was Turi Josefsen (born 1936 in Hammerfest, Norway). Turi is a Norwegian-American businesswoman. She was Vice-President of United States Surgical Corporation (USSC) (headed by her ex-husband, Leon C Hirsch), and CEO of the European division, Auto Suture Europe. In the early 1990s, she was the highest-paid woman in corporate America and at one time reportedly the world's highest paid woman CEO. When they separated, Turi took over the running of Europe – probably so they didn't clash – while Leon stayed in Norwalk at HQ. His car was regularly checked for bombs and his security was always tight after threats against his life from the extreme animal activists.

After USSC was taken over by Tyco International, she joined the board of WebSurg S.A., a pioneering online surgical training programme.

Turi Josefsen has invested considerably in the Hammerfest area, including part-funding a new equestrian centre in 2003 and extending the small local runway to accommodate her private jet. She published a book and commissioned a film about the region. Turi has endowed fellowships and chairs in surgery, including a Chair of Surgery at the University of Illinois at Chicago (UIC).

When I was employed as a Regional Sales Director for Vascular Therapies (A new division of USSC Auto Suture), I spent a lot of time at Elancourt near Paris. It was known as Turi's Taj Mahal as no expense had been spared in her design of the European office and training centre. When I was promoted into this RSD position, Turi would often call me at home – always at night – and always late at night. Her work patterns meant when she wanted to talk to you, she called. Family life did not come into it. USSC divorce rate was also one of the highest in the industry.

Lots of water under the bridge, but in 2013 I had dinner with Turi and an old colleague Charles Reynolds in Paris. She was not scary at all anymore. In fact, she was charming. We dined at the Bristol Hotel in Paris which was one of her favourites. Like me, she is recovering from cancer – breast cancer in her case and we talked about all sorts. She was going to pick up the bill but I insisted on paying. I said "Turi, the training and business development I experienced at USSC prepared me for all my future successes. Please allow me to pay for dinner".

One of the key roles an experienced Product Specialist for Auto Suture could fulfil was helping the Management recruit new sales people. Usually, there was 4 or 5 interviews plus a psychometric test. If the potential candidate got through those stages, he was then asked to go into Theatre (OR) to make sure they could cope with that unique environment. The investment of a 6-week residential course in Norwalk Connecticut was a big one for the Auto Suture Corporation. Therefore, no stone was left unturned before flights were booked and the candidate was sent on the gruelling training course. Many people did not make it. They were either sent home − with no job − or they left of their own accord. Not good for either the company or the candidate.

After a couple of years in the role I was asked to meet a chap called David Frederick. I made arrangements to meet him in the Hospital café of the Southern General Hospital Glasgow (now the Queen Elizabeth University Hospital) at 8am. When I arrived, David was tucking into two "rolls and sausage". I found this a little surprising and asked him if he had been in Theatre (OR) before. I got a single syllable answer "no" as he continued his assault on the greasy sausage rolls. First impressions!?

I took him into the changing rooms for the Operating Suites. I showed him how to get dressed into theatre greens, put on his mask and cap, theatre clogs etc. I also told him what he was about to experience. Informed him about the sterile field and warned him if he felt in any way faint, he should walk away, and whatever he did, NOT to fall forwards towards the patient if he felt himself "going". Not unusual for a first time. I said I would be right behind him. Anyway, I could tell David thought I was an idiot and being too precious in my preparation of him.

We were in the Southern General Hospital in Glasgow where I had undergone my own introduction to the OR. It was an old Victorian hospital and with two surgeons I knew well: Graham Sunderland and Ross Carter – both General Surgeons who used staple guns and who were pioneering the Laparoscopic boom at that time, which was exploding globally, for minimally invasive surgery. As well as supplying the surgical staple devices, we also had some of the best trocars, hand instruments and clip devices for Laparoscopic surgery.

The first case was a full laparotomy for a bowel resection which involved cutting through the abdomen with the use of scalpels and electro cautery to stop any bleeding. This produces a lot of smell also – of burning flesh. A theatre nurse asked me a question and I engaged with her for a second. When I turned back, David was gone. In a split second, he had scampered off, opened the window in the operating room – a BIG no no – and was "heaving" out of the window.

I was horrified. The surgeons stopped, looked up and I think it was Graham Sunderland who said "first time?" I apologised profusely and said "yes". I went and got David, closed the window and left the operating room. I sat him down and got him some water. That could have been it for David, his potential Auto Suture career could have been over right there. However, having spent so long in sales and sales recruitment something inside me was saying "this guy's got something".

The next case was a Laparoscopic Cholecystectomy. It was a minimally invasive case and would not involve cutting, scalpels and burning flesh smells. So I prepared him, told him what he was about to see and about 2 hours later, we were in the operating room again.

The way David tells the story now is much funnier than I can write it. He recalls seeing this "old fella being wheeled in and a needle being stuck into his belly button, the gas insufflation through the needle pumped his stomach up before the main scope trocar/port was rammed in". A trocar is basically an extremely sharp cutting punch around 10mms in diameter. It's a medical device that is made up of an obturator (which may be a metal or plastic sharpened or non-bladed tip), a cannula (basically a hollow tube), and a seal. Trocars are placed through the abdomen during laparoscopic surgery. The trocar functions as a portal for the subsequent placement of other instruments, such as graspers, scissors, staplers, etc. It's basically pushed with some force through the wall of the abdomen and the cutting element is removed.

That was enough. David was off again feeling sick. At least this time he scampered out of the operating room to the waiting area to catch his breath.

As I said, there was something about him. I told the management I liked him, and a week later David was off to the USA for 6 weeks. He not only became one of the most successful Product Specialists in the company, but over a number of years, he rose to the level of Vice President. David and I became friends outside of work and we are still good friends.

Since then, David has started his own distribution company called HC21 along with Owen Curtin in the UK and Ireland. Within two years, their turnover was over £60 million per annum due to some clever contracts he negotiated with Covidien and other large medical corporations. He is Chairman of Alesi-Surgical also, and Alesi is one of my clients (story coming). As you will see, many people from my past keep coming back.

David asked me to get involved to do what I do best: build distribution and sales of Ultravision – a device for clearing the visual field during Laparoscopic Surgery. Clever piece of kit. A classic **Idea in Medicine.**

Best of Health

In 1998, as previously mentioned, Tyco Healthcare bought USSC (Auto Suture) in a number of large acquisitions they made in that year.

I was the Regional Sales Director of the Vascular Therapies division at that time and was offered two choices. The first was a lucrative redundancy package, and the second was to be moved back into one of the other Divisions as Tyco intended to merge the Vascular Therapies division back into the core business. I decided to take the generous package and left. I was not quite sure what I wanted to do, but for sure I would look to develop a business of some sort.

The friend I mentioned earlier, Ramsay McLellan, had come across a cervical screening opportunity and he asked my advice. We looked at this closely, and little was I to know what this would lead to. It was a strange business in many ways but we saw growth potential, as there had been a number of high-profile media campaigns highlighting the need for women to have easier access to this type of screening. It was at that time we approached a mutual friend of ours, Bert Jukes, about the business. He rightly spotted a number of flaws in the business model and convinced us to walk away. The ground was set for us to do some sort of business together.

Bert is a larger-than-life character who was the first person to get me on my feet public speaking. I used to hate the thought of public speaking to the point of being physically sick. During my wedding reception, I couldn't even eat my meal as I was so nervous. We made the mistake of having the speeches after dinner. Bert had me public speaking at meetings every week and it has grown to be one of my strengths.

Whoever heard of a salesman who had a fear of public speaking? Well it happens. It was me! I have learned a lot from Bert over the years.

Bert was and is a great public speaker. He is a natural and has a great sense of humour. He loves making people laugh and he is good at it. Bert is a big family man and his wife Faye is a great support for Bert. His kids Steven, David Alan and Gillian are a credit to Bert and Faye. He has watched my two grow up and I have seen the same with Bert's.

New projects are currently developing with Bert and I, involving one of my Icelandic clients – exciting times ahead.

Around that time, my wife had been invited to a Sunday lunch with a family in Milngavie, on the outskirts of Glasgow. Dr Greg Steiner was an Osteopath and he had an extensive library. I had a good look through his collection and was drawn to a book by Professor Brian Peskin called Radiant Health. I borrowed the book and was fascinated by its content. This controversial, outspoken Professor, was one of the first exposures I had to the benefits of nutrition and especially of Omega3. Most of the work I had been doing in the medical industry to that point had been treating people after they had become ill. It really appealed to me to help develop an educational programme to stop people becoming ill in the first place. So I re-read the book and made direct contact with Professor Peskin who was an MIT graduate and Professor. I then told Bert and Ramsay there was a great business opportunity involved. I flew to Houston to meet Professor Peskin and he very kindly spent the weekend discussing his scientific and research findings. He was delighted that his work was attracting international attention and recognition.

There it was: with my partners, Bert Jukes and Ramsay McLellan, Best of Health was born, and we set about helping people control their health and weight with an educational programme and supplements. It was an Idea in Medicine from outside mainstream but a hugely popular alternative route which millions of people have an interest in.

The business built great momentum very quickly and Bert, Ramsay and I successfully launched in the UK and then developed further afield into Italy, France, Germany and Scandinavia. Bert went to live in the USA and took control of the business there. It was an education on many fronts. We learned as much about how not to run a business, as how to successfully run a business. We all learned many lessons and made a number of strategic mistakes which ultimately cost us. However, what we learned about the benefits of nutrition and Omega3 have stayed with me to this day.

We were really ahead of the nutritional game with Best of Health, and at the time, our message was not always enthusiastically accepted. We were very aware that the right kind of fat was good for you, whereas back then, dietary fat was the bad guy. Also, the whole issue of processed carbs and protein in our message was again…. ahead of the game. We were very good at our education though, and many sports personalities got on board. Sam Torrance and almost half of his Ryder Cup team that won at the Belfry were on our programme. John Parrot and many other snooker players also. One of the elements was that concentration could be helped by ensuring your Omega 3 levels were appropriate.

Eventually, we even developed a blood test to check a person's Omega 3 levels and this was conducted personally by a "finger stick" and swab and the analysis was done at Stirling University. This university was famous for its work on Omega 3.

I still supplement with Omega3 and Ramsay developed the brand I prefer after I left the Best of Health. He called it "Ideal Omega" and this brand is recognised internationally as one of the best in the world. It has the highest and purest levels of EPA and DHA which is where the benefits of Omega 3 come from. In fact, the success of his brand grew enormously and his own Ideas in Medicine, Healthy and Essential, was sold to Dermasalve PLC in 2006. He eventually bought the brand back in 2009. Ramsay had ensured he had all the trademarks, domain names etc. which gave him options about the best way to sell.

Medicapro and the Oil Industry

Following The Best of Health, I formed a company called Medicapro Ltd and partnered with a strong team, David Frederick, Paul Blenkinsopp and Alex Bonthrone. I had worked with all the guys at Auto Suture and we knew each other very well.

We formed the company and then looked around for opportunities. We started trading in certain sectors which did not result in quick sales. Then we were contacted by a business called GX Laboratories run by a businessman called Tim Rogers. They needed help expanding into the medical sector and we were recommended to them. Talk about a character! Although we had started negotiations with another of the company's directors, Tim got back from vacation and called me. His exact words were "you have been dealing with the monkeys and I am the organ grinder!!" Tim was, and is, a real character, unique, and we have had some intense experiences together – but also some real fun.

So we thrashed out a deal and we quickly helped Tim and his business expand. GX Laboratories was formed to develop a unique biocide called G-Cide. The need for effective biocides was clear as the MRSA (Methicillin-resistant Staphylococcus aureus) scare had really impacted the Hospital systems globally. The UK was particularly badly hit by MRSA. We started helping a South African scientist called Toni Martin who developed G-Cide to get her message across. and We assisted GX Laboratories in their approach to the Hospital Units and Medical Device Distributors Internationally.

At this point, another business lesson kicked in. GX Laboratories were raising money and they brought in some VC investors who changed the dynamic of the business. If ever a lesson needed to be learned about the price you will pay if you accept your funding from a wrong source, this was it. The new board of GX transformed after the money was accepted, and they turned from an exciting fun venture with people who worked well together into a company where promises meant very little and the desire for control and power was all.

They collapsed of course, and Medicapro Ltd was one of the victims. We had put our full effort into building sales through GX Labs and we felt our contract was solid. Another one of the victims was my "organ grinder" pal Tim Rogers who had been turned into one of the monkeys. He was deeply unhappy at what had transpired and had done everything possible to protect Medicapro Ltd. We all ended up being shoved aside as the Investor Group took control. It gives me no satisfaction to say that they subsequently failed and the company went into liquidation. They had no experience in the Medical sector and their desire to get the products to consumers failed.

The relationship between Tim and myself has flourished however. Even stronger now because of the challenges. Our families know each other, we have been on holidays together and we speak every week. It was because of my relationship with Tim that a significant non-medical project has developed.

Tim got busy after GX Laboratories, and his strong relationships with Dow Chemicals and background with Flow Laboratories helped him develop a unique product. Working with chemists we knew, Tim had a hunch that there was a sector of the oil industry that was not serviced by existing companies. Along with his brother Mark, we formed an oil company.

We developed a product which "thins" heavy oil and cleans up paraffin plugs often created in oil wells. Steam was, and is being used, which is ecologically unfriendly, expensive and only works temporarily.

A unique soy-based compound was created which clears the plugs and thins oil. Totem Oil was born. Our first investor was my brother-in-law Barney Raku-Eavns who has been in the oil industry all his life after he left the army. We think of him as a proper oil man. Tim's brother Mark has been a major part in the company's structure and success. Mark is a great balance for the character of Tim, and together, they make a great team. I help with introductions and advice, and the nice thing about the oil industry is that you can add zeros very easily in this enormous sector. Oil is one of the largest business sectors in the world, and it's great to be a part of it.

Since then, the business has expanded into Asia, the Middle East and the USA. Dr Eyad (more on Dr Eyad later) became a major partner through my introductions, and the business is expanding rapidly. With the oil price currently very low, it's even more important to get oil out of the ground economically. So, once again, relationships are providing the basis of this business success and its current growth. It's almost a mantra to keep my friends and colleagues close.

Breaking Stones

Paul Molloy is another close friend and business colleague and we go way back. Where did we meet? The Vascular Therapies Division (as mentioned previously part of USSC) was about to go through a restructure and Bob Knarr (part of the USSC founding team) who was President of USSC and a senior director set up a meeting with the directors of the Division to implement the "restructuring" of Vascular Therapies. Of the four Regional Sales Directors, we knew two were being fired – we just didn't know which two. Being one of the four, I was a little nervous, although I remember being quietly confident I would be fine as my sales were the best. I remember Paul and I preparing for the presentation to Bob. Paul was brilliantly confident. His attitude was very much "we are great and if you let us go, it's your loss". I loved it.

Anyway, after an expensive dinner at the Frankfurt Sheraton – a hotel I have used since many times - the next day unfolded with the usual tension. The French and Italian Regional Sales Directors were fired, and myself and the German RSD were retained along with Paul as the Marketing Director.

The medical device industry is truly amazing as even since I started to prepare and write this book over 6 months ago, Bob Knarr is now back in my life. He has just been appointed as CEO and a board member for Mederi Inc., one of my most important clients, and Will Rutan (story coming) asked him to bring his vast experience to the table to help us grow.

I played golf with Bob and Will in June 2015 in Blue Hill Maine at an event hosted by Will and his family to commemorate both his parents who died within a short time of each other. Tough year for Will. I had a real laugh with Bob as I recounted the Frankfurt experience over one of his famously expensive bottles of red wine which he loves.

Anyway, I digress. Paul is currently the CEO at ClearFlow Inc., a medical device industry start-up headquartered in Southern California and focused on commercializing a patented post-surgical wound management system for the prevention of Retained Blood Complications.

In May 2006, Paul asked me to join him at LMA Urology (story coming). Paul is a classic guy. He started off in marketing and is an Ideas in Medicine visionary in many ways. Paul is a cup-half-full kind of guy. He sees the potential always before the challenges. I have always liked working with Paul. He has been a big influence on me and the role in LMA came through him. My early support of ClearFlow was because of his approach for my help to build sales internationally.

Prior to ClearFlow, he worked with the current investors of ClearFlow at VasoNova Inc. a Silicon Valley based and venture-funded vascular ultrasound navigation technology acquired by Teleflex Inc. in January 2011. He was appointed President of Teleflex's largest division after he successfully merged VasoNova into the vascular division with full P&L responsibility for direct sales, US and overseas manufacturing plants, R&D and strategic planning at a corporate level.

Paul has over twenty years' experience of public, private and VC funded medical device companies. He is a Board member at two medical device companies presently, and was a Board member at LMA and VasoNova, including European and Asian subsidiaries.

Paul took LMA public in 2005 and it was acquired by Teleflex in 2012 in a process he brokered. Paul was a practicing Certified Registered Nurse Anaesthetist until joining Datascope Corp in NJ in 1989, obtaining his MBA from the University of Chicago's Booth School of Business and managing through successive executive positions with leading medical device firms. He has extensive global industry connections and has travelled, lived and worked in Europe, Asia and the USA, including substantial experience setting up and managing operations in many of these countries as well as serving on the Board of these companies. He currently lives in Southern California – which he loves.

He is an experienced CEO & General Manger. He also has Board-level skills and is on the board at ClearFlow Inc. and Creative Vascular Inc. Paul has significant public company investor environment management and private equity and venture capital relationships.

Even as I writing this, I am thinking Paul should be a board member of Ideas in Medicine Ltd. He has classic experience spanning a couple of decades now. I recently approached Paul about a new tracheostomy device–and so this story is ongoing.

One of the most charismatic characters I met during this period was Dr Markus Haller. I met Marcus during a dinner in Lausanne, Switzerland, along with Robert Gaines-Cooper and his wife. Robert is a Seychelles-based billionaire and has taken a number of unique **Ideas in Medicine** to profitable fruition. We had dinner in the famous Beau-Rivage Spa Hotel on the shores of Lake Geneva in Lausanne. Robert wanted me to meet Markus who he was considering appointing as CEO of LMA Urology. I liked Markus immediately. A cowboy boot-wearing German who has properties in Switzerland and Boulder, Colarado. Markus was another who had cut his teeth in Medtronic and then gone on to successfully manage start-ups in the medical device industry.

When we met, HMRC were trying to make Robert Gaines £30 million poorer, after the Court of Appeal ruled that the Her Majesties Revenues and Customs (HMRC) were justified in considering whether he had properly severed his links with the UK. This was when assessing whether he was a UK resident for the purposes of paying tax. Robert was, amazingly, very relaxed about all that and he subsequently won the appeal and HMRC had to settle for a more modest £600,000 payment.

Robert is based in the Seychelles and, on average, has not spent longer than 91 days a year in the UK since 1976. However, he has a house in Henley-on-Thames, his son was educated in an English school, he is a regular at Ascot, he often spends Christmas in the UK and his will was drawn up under English law. All of this led HMRC to believe that Mr Gaines-Cooper did not qualify for exemptions from British taxes as a non-resident. Anyway, HMRC brought a case which could have seriously affected many ex pats with British backgrounds.

Anyway, Robert asked me what I thought of Marcus after the dinner and I said. "Hire him". Markus is a results-orientated, no-nonsense, direct personality. Exactly what we needed in LMA at that time. I knew he would ruffle feathers and he did, but I loved working with him and learned a lot.

For a couple of years, we travelled the world together building the LMA Urology start-up business. Professor Rane who I wrote about earlier was on our Scientific Advisory Board and he and I travelled extensively also.

The LMA StoneBreaker is a portable, non-electrical, compact intracorporeal lithotripter, intended for use to fragment stones in the urinary tract (i.e. kidney, ureter and bladder). It weighs around 500g with a probe and it requires no extraneous electrical or pneumatic connections. It is a great and simple device and I loved building the business.

The StoneBreaker carbon dioxide (CO_2) gas cartridge typically provides the necessary energy for one surgical procedure.

So in June 2009, a deal was struck between LMA and Cook Medical. I am excited to say that I set the deal up. I approached Cook's Senior VP Jerry French and explained why I thought the Stonebreaker would be a good fit for their Urology Division. Jerry agreed and so the due diligence commenced. It was at that time one of my most memorable business trips took place. I had a number of key meetings to prepare the ground for the deal so here was my 10-day flight path.

Glasgow, London, Bangkok, Singapore, Melbourne, Auckland, Los Angeles, Dallas, Raleigh Durham and then back to Glasgow via London. I have been travelling globally for many years, but that was literally a trip which circumnavigated the globe.

Markus was great and I thoroughly enjoyed participating in the negotiations. I learned a lot from the experience. Here is part of the news release

"Cook Medical and LMA Urology Ltd have entered into a strategic partnership that can significantly improve the remedies available for stone disease management. Through the worldwide agreement, Cook will market and distribute LMA's StoneBreaker™, a portable pneumatic, endoscopic lithotripter for stone fragmentation. StoneBreaker is a powerful, easy-to-manage and cost-effective lithotripter, and will be marketed in conjunction with Cook's own cutting-edge portfolio of stone management technologies and devices. Together, they provide urologists across the globe with a highly effective, end-to-end solution for treating kidney, ureteral and bladder stones, reducing procedure times and improving overall patient care.

The LMA StoneBreaker is a proprietary device that is highly effective in the treatment of urinary stone disease. The StoneBreaker's unique, compact, ergonomic design makes it easier to manage than comparable lithotripters, reducing the procedure time for fragmentation and removal of stones. Additionally, there is minimal probe movement during the procedure allowing for safer stone fragmentation and reduced stone migration. Powered by a cartridge of high-pressure carbon dioxide gas, the StoneBreaker delivers a higher probe-tip velocity at impact to successfully break stones in one procedure, thus eliminating the need for additional costly procedure time and patient discomfort.

Dr. Demetrius Bagley, the Nathan Lewis Hatfield Professor of Urology at Thomas Jefferson University, Jefferson Medical Center and an internationally recognized expert in endourology, has recently concluded a study on use of the StoneBreaker. He notes, "The StoneBreaker has a number of advantages. It is comfortable to use, portable and relatively inexpensive compared to other types of endoscopic lithotripters. Used with a rigid endoscope, the probe provides excellent stone fragmentation. The stone starts breaking with minimal migration. Unlike laser lithotripters, the StoneBreaker requires no special team to perform the procedure."

Commenting on the Cook Medical partnership, Dr. Markus Haller, president of LMA Urology said, "We are delighted to have Cook Medical as our partner. The company's vast expertise in urology, combined with its substantial marketing and sales capability will allow us to achieve global market penetration for the StoneBreaker. Together, our companies provide today's urologists with a comprehensive solution for stone management."

"We are very excited to be working with LMA, a company that continues to demonstrate product excellence and quality-focused innovation in treatment of stone disorders," said Jerry French, senior vice president and global strategic business leader for Cook Medical's urology division. "Together, we offer an industry-leading stone management technology that provides urologists worldwide with a more comprehensive approach to treat kidney, ureteral and bladder stones, minimizing procedure time and improving overall patient care."

This was major milestone for me in helping pull such a deal together. It was very rewarding and satisfying.

Sophono

In 2007, as previously mentioned, I was introduced to Dr Markus Haller by Robert Gaines Cooper. Markus and I have kept in touch ever since. Markus is certainly in "play" right now as an Executive who can take start-up businesses and get them to exit for the benefit of the shareholders and investors.

In June 2009, Markus founded Sophono Inc. with the ambitious goal to improve the lives of patients with bone conduction hearing loss. At that time, the only real option for those patients was the BAHA product, with a constantly infected skin-penetrating screw on which an external sound processor was mounted.

Markus's investment company Windgan Holding SA invested as initial Angel Investor into Sophono. In 2010 Sophono acquired Otomag GmbH a company primarily owned by Prof. Ralf Siegert, who was the medical inventor of the Sophono device and had already implanted it into the first 100 patients at that time.

In July 2010, Sophono received ISO 13485 certification and prepared the full 510k submission to FDA. In May 2011 Sophono received FDA clearance to market the world's first transcutaneous bone conduction hearing implant system, this was the beginning of the end of the then current percutaneous devices.

In 2012, Sophono raised US $7M from Wexford Capital, a US-based VC, to begin full commercialization on the product – and is now represented in over 45 countries. Further investments were obtained finally adding up to a total of $14M. In 2013, Dr. Peter Ruppersberg joined the company as CEO, while Sophono remained under the overall direction of the founding Chairman Dr. Markus Haller. As you can see, Markus has all the experience necessary to bring a project from conception to commercialisation.

By the end of 2014, Sophono had achieved over 4,000 patients world-wide. Finally, in the summer of 2014, initial discussions with strategic partners were started, and eventually, in March 2015, Dr. Markus Haller's first employer announced the acquisition of Sophono Inc. and the integration of the company into its ENT business.

So guess who bought Sophono? That's right, our friends at Medtronic. Its fascinating to me how Medtronic has featured in so many of the companies I have worked for!

I never worked for them directly, but it feels as though I have!

Tenaxis

Following the offloading of LMA Stonebreaker to Cook, I was then looking for my next role. I was offered a role within the established LMA mask business but it didn't feel quite me. The role of Distributor Management was similar to what I had being doing except that the business was well-established. The excitement of the start-up was gone. I love building things whereas the role within the mask division meant handling a declining business. The patents had expired and the Chinese in particular had flooded the market with numerous copies – less expensive of course. LMA were performing an admirable job in holding back the tide, but slowly and surely, market share was being eroded.

I was called up by a Headhunter and he described a role which seemed perfect. An American start up called Tenaxis Medical was looking for a global Sales and Marketing Director. They had developed a surgical sealant to stop bleeding following operations such as coronary artery bypass (CABG), vascular procedures etc. The product was called ArterX Vascular Sealant

ArterX Vascular Sealant is a novel prophylactic agent that seals anastomotic suture lines in seconds. The sealant quickly sets into a soft gel that contains a unique cross-linking agent to provide strong covalent bonding between tissues and effectively seals grafts. ArterX requires no mixing, is easy to apply and is effective in both wet and dry fields.

The product seemed ideal, the company seemed ideal and after meeting the CEO at the Sofitel in Terminal 5 Heathrow, it was clear David Smith thought I was ideal. Following the meeting, he flew me out to San Francisco to meet the founder Ron Diek. Ron is a serial entrepreneur and had already established and sold a number of innovative medical devices. Ron had already had three successful **Ideas in Medicine** which he had sold for multi millions of dollars.

Ron is another classic example of a person who creatively thinks up product ideas and gets them to market. Ron's game plan though, as evidenced by other projects he has been involved in, is the "build to sell" model. He has his eureka moment, goes through patent protections, sets his company up around it, invests in product development, registrations, regulatory, commercialises to prove concept and then sells his company to the highest bidder. Classic **Ideas in Medicine** in motion.

Tenaxis Medical Inc. were based in Menlo Park outside San Francisco where many US start-ups begin their Life. In fact, Google was a few blocks down. I got on well with all the staff and started to prepare myself. The offer was excellent, including a motivating share option offer, and I was excited about the role and the product. I started to grow sales aggressively and do what I had been brought on to do – develop the business.

We had a booth at the European Association of Cardio Thoracic Surgery - which in 2009 was in Vienna. David Smith said he was coming over and bringing a staff member Leslie Reno who was helping with their pivotal Food and Drug Association (FDA) study which they needed for approval to sell in the USA. The Food and Drug Administration (FDA or USFDA) is a federal agency of the United States Department of Health and Human Services, one of the United States federal executive departments. It is a hard nut to crack for new medical devices and becoming harder. To gain access to the world's biggest economy, you have to jump through a few hoops. This is one of the key elements of Ideas in Medicine as we have the contacts and expertise to help navigate the FDA, CE and BRIC (Brazil, Russia, India and China) registrations.

The FDA is responsible for protecting and promoting public health through the regulation and supervision of food safety, tobacco products, dietary supplements, prescription and over-the-counter pharmaceutical drugs (medications), vaccines, biopharmaceuticals, blood transfusions, medical devices, electromagnetic radiation emitting devices (ERED), cosmetics, animal foods & feed and veterinary products.

We had a CE mark to sell in the European Union. The CE mark, or formerly EC mark, is a mandatory conformity marking for certain products sold within the European Economic Area (EEA) since 1985. The CE marking is also found on products sold outside the EEA that are manufactured in, or designed to be sold in, the EEA. This makes the CE marking recognizable worldwide even to people who are not familiar with the European Economic Area. It is in that sense similar to the FCC Declaration of Conformity used on certain electronic devices sold in the United States. It consists of the CE logo and, if applicable, the four-digit identification number of the notified body involved in the conformity assessment procedure. The CE marking is the manufacturer's declaration that the product meets the requirements of the applicable EC directives.

The actual words signified by "CE" have been disputed. It is often taken to be an abbreviation of Conformité Européenne, meaning "European Conformity". However, "CE" originally stood for "Communauté Européenne", French for "European Community". In former German legislation, the CE marking was called "EG-Zeichen" meaning "European Community mark". The CE marking is a symbol of free marketability in the European Economic Area (Internal Market), therefore, a great first move for most start-ups. It is likewise generally easier than obtaining FDA approval. Also, the CE mark makes it possible to sell in the Middle East and many other parts of the world.

Anyway, back to the Tenaxis story, we were all meeting up at Heathrow and David and Lesley had just got off a flight from San Francisco. I flew down from Glasgow and we were all on the same BA flight to Vienna. I offered to take them into the BA lounge to freshen up.

Things started really well and some key distributors were brought on board. I had built a strong friendship with Stavros Vizirgianakis in South Africa. He was another ex USSC (Auto Suture) manager. In fact, he had been GM for South Africa. Stavros and I met in Dubai at Arab Health and he loved Arterx and believed he could make quick inroads into selling the product.

Stavros works closely with his brother Greg Vizirgianakis – who is a neuro surgeon. We had organised a distributor management meeting in St Andrews, Scotland. By that time, Stavros was a board member and we were all very positive about how we could expand the use of ArterX in surgery internationally. Greg came over to the event and it was a terrific focus meeting with Greg lending his surgical expertise to the discussions and helping the other distributors understand why the sealant was so good. Not only that, but the international guests loved St Andrews. Who wouldn't?

For various different reasons – including recovery from my cancer – I stopped working as an employee for Tenaxis Medical in 2011.

Ron took over the day-to-day running of his company in 2012 and then asked if I could work with them again. I did so, but not as an employee. It suited me to work as a Consultant for them, which was the start of my current business path. Life is amazing. I was happy that Ron and the management team asked for my help once I got "on the road" again.

The Tenaxis share option package become very valuable as about a year later, Ron and the board sold Tenaxis Medical to The Medicine's Company of Parsippany, New Jersey and I made a tidy sum from the sale.

The Tenaxis story was one of the most impactful in my life for good and bad reasons. When I look back, it seems almost unbelievable. However, let's not forget it is a classic Ideas in Medicine story.

So from that point, I worked with Tenaxis again as a Consultant and then was rapidly offered roles with Bionova in Australia (which sold to LeMaitre) and Pluromed in the USA (which sold to Sanofi Biosurgery). It was a totally incredible time. I had already started consulting with Mederi Therapeutics (story coming) in the USA just after my recovery. Mederi remain to this day one of my most important clients. The connections again are obvious, and when you deliver results and do a good job, you get noticed.

Meanwhile, the Vizirgianakis brothers have been busy, and recently, Greg called me with a new project.

DISA Vascular is an innovative medical device company that specialises in vascular technology for the treatment of coronary artery disease (CAD). www.disavascular.com Situated in Cape Town, South Africa, the company has been developing stents for the international market since its inception in 1998, and in the process realising its vision of *Bringing Quality to Life*.

Through in-depth research and development, and a total commitment to patient care, the company has produced high-quality medical devices. Today, their products are sold via a network of distributors in many parts of the world and through their direct sales force in all cardiac hospitals in South Africa.

DISA Vascular has EN ISO 9001, EN ISO 13485 and MDD93/42/EEC certifications. All the products carry the European CE mark and have also gained regulatory approval in various other regions of the world. The company's CEO is a gentleman called Markus Lehmann. Markus has ensured German quality standards in all manufacturing processes. They have asked if I will head their international sales management and expansion. New products are coming and existing lines are being advanced. Very exciting as I know the standards of the people involved and I have a history with them.

The Big C

It's often possible to look back and marvel when life throws you some unexpected shocks. In 2012, I was travelling back from San Antonio in Texas from the Society of American Gastrointestinal and Endoscopic Surgeons (SAGES) meeting. What I was doing at this Congress will become clear in later chapters. I am actually editing these chapters in San Antonio Texas in March 2016. I am here for Distributor training event with a client Hovertech (story to come) Heading to SAGES in Boston next week. How strange and connected life can be.

Anyway, in 2012, I was in a BA flat bed and during the overnight flight, I felt an uncomfortable sensation, not really a pain, in my privates. I went to the doctor and he sent me for a scan. I watched the reaction of the young sonographer and saw her face when she was scanning me. I asked her what she had found and she said "I can't say but you need to go back to your GP tomorrow". I knew then something wasn't right.

I went back to the doctor's surgery in Killearn and a young GP was the doctor I had to see. I found out I had cancer when I was handed a sheet that said "How to Cope with Cancer"! I don't think things had sunk in when he said "I am sending you to Dr. so and so (can't remember the name) at Stirling Royal Infirmary tomorrow". I was more than a little agitated and said "no you are not, give me an hour".

As you will read shortly, my path is soon heading towards my entry into the medical world. Following my stint as a Recruitment Consultant, I saw an advertisement for a Medical Device Rep. This immediately rang a bell remembering all those smart young reps I would see when I was working as a hospital porter. I loved the fact this resonated from those first days of getting myself sorted out. I applied and got the job (storyline to come). My experience in the medical device world was about to get fast tracked.

Back to my illness. One of the advantages of working in the medical industry is that we know there are different standards everywhere. That includes, surgeons, nurses, support staff etc. We know the good surgeons and we especially know the bad ones. To be fair, I didn't know the Urologist the young GP was referring me to, but I knew a friend who did. I left the surgery and called Abhay Rane.

Professor Abhay Rane is a Urologist I have known for many years. In fact, to give him his full title, it's Professor Abhay Rane, OBE, MS, FRCS (Urol). Professor Rane was appointed an Officer of the Order of the British Empire in the New Year 2014 Honours List for services to laparoscopic urology. Professor Rane has been a Consultant Urological Surgeon at Surrey and Sussex NHS Trust for the last 14 years, where he is currently Clinical Lead for urology.

He is one of the first laparoscopic urological surgeons in the United Kingdom. Instrumental in developing the technique of hand assisted laparoscopic nephrectomy in the UK from 2000, he was the first to describe the usefulness of the technique in T3b (advanced) kidney cancers. More recently, he spearheaded the development of laparo- endoscopic single site surgery (LESS) in Urology as a pioneer and innovator. Having performed the first single port nephrectomy in the world in May 2007 with colleagues in India, he went on to perform the first LESS nephrectomy in Europe in March 2008 at East Surrey Hospital.

Over the last twelve years, Professor Rane has mentored laparoscopic skills to many other consultants. As a result of his efforts, at least 16 hospitals in the UK now have a local laparoscopic urology programs; his work on training in laparoscopy has been presented, published and cited extensively. So I count myself very fortunate that I can call on surgeons like Abhay for advice. In fact, Abhay and I have travelled the word together during the LMA

Stonebreaker project (storyline to come). Abhay was on the Scientific Advisory Board for LMA on the Stonebreaker project

Abhay was incredibly helpful, and I will be for ever grateful for his immediate guidance. He told me where I needed to go and who I had to see. He referred me to a surgeon called Mr Khurram Mir at the Southern General Hospital (now the magnificent Queen Elizabeth University Hospital). Abhay is English from an Indian ethnicity and Kurram Mir from a Pakistan ethnicity – and we all know there is no love lost between those countries. I knew this Surgeon must be good.

In fact, that same day, he called his ex-colleague Khurram and asked if he would see me. Mr Mir said he was operating that day but he would see me between patients. I went along to the Theatre (Operating Room or OR) and waited. As soon as I walked in, one of the senior nurses recognised me and said "Graeme, hi, what are you doing here?"

I was a little cautious. Concerned that Mr Mir may have gotten into a little bother as some Theatre Managers are tough as nails. As he came out of the OR, he said "Nurse hi, I am seeing Graeme up in my private offices" and she said "No, you are not, you can see Graeme here. Let me prepare an examination table for him".   Again, it's sometimes who you know in these situations!

He physically examined me and said he did not feel anything unusual but he needed to see the scan. So my hopes went sky high because truth be told, I always felt "Cancer, me, surely not???". I am sure many people have experienced the same.

Anyway, next morning he called and –boom- I was floored again as he said I had Stage 1 Seminoma and would need my left testicle surgically removed immediately to ensure the cancer wouldn't spread! Oh boy, I had always thought testicular cancer was a young man's cancer. In fact, the Oncologists later did say I was at the upper end of the age they had ever seen this cancer.

The next day, I was booked into Ross Hall Hospital and the procedure was done. I was in the Theatre (OR) where I had often worked and been supporting procedures and now there I was, surrounded by staff who knew me by first name (you'll see why a little later in the book), about to go under the scalpel. The procedure went well and I was sent home with a ton of Tramadol for the pain and antibiotics to prevent infection.

The next question I had to deal with was the Chemotherapy. It's usually a choice, never a must, and again I spoke with some surgeon pals to seek advice. One of whom had also had testicular cancer. I had the chemo.

Yuk! Not nice. The Beatson Clinic in Glasgow is an excellent facility and the staff have been incredibly supportive. I was now in the system. Every three months for the first three years, I went for blood tests and X-Rays. I have now moved on to check-ups every 6 months and all is clear! You have no idea how good that sounds when you hear those words "all clear" when you have had a cancer. As I write this on a Wednesday, my next check-up is Friday and so I am always a little nervous.

I am constantly aware now, and all the ads on TV for cancer charities have a more meaningful impact. However, I move on. I try to eat well, keep myself fit and active. I still have bad days and down days like everybody else, but I am more appreciative of life in general.

From my early twenties after getting my life back in order, I have made a significant effort to be the best I can be. I spend a lot of time reading and listening to self-development material.

When your system gets a shock and you are told you have cancer, then the hours spent exploring self-development concepts become very valuable. I have become very selective over the years and only a few of the self-development people still resonate with me. The recently deceased Jim Rohn was good to read and listen to on his "philosophy of life" approach.

On a practical level and from a sales point of view, Jeffrey Gitomer and his very focussed sales material is always good value. I worked with Jeffrey during future business projects such as The Best of Health (storyline later)–I remember attending a training day he did for the Financial Times Advertising Sales Staff in the City of London. The hard-nosed big city advertising sales guys were totally spellbound by Jeffrey's no-nonsense sales approach. My son-in-law Max was given a copy of Jeffrey's book "The Sales Bible". Max reckons this helped him become one of the top sales people in the branch. This was Max's first job in sales for PC World. Max has since moved on after two years to an excellent Computer Tech support role for a major British company.

Anyway, the London Financial Times day was great and as well as learning a lot I had great fun. We then jumped on a train and went up to Leeds where he was helping to train some of our Sales Agents for The Best of Health. Find some of Jeffrey's material on www.gitomer.com

I also spent a number of years using a meditation system of binaural beats called Holosync developed by a Californian (go figure) called Bill Harris. It's been great while travelling as basically all you do is put headphones

101

on and relax. The recording does the rest and has been scientifically proven to take you to deep meditative levels without using mantras or worrying about what thoughts are moving through your head. Bill also has an amazing philosophy of life and I have been on his courses and taken his online trainings. These have helped during some of my hardest stressful times.

Also, Jordon Belfort of Wolf of Wall Street fame has been fascinating me. His crazy and amazing life in Wall Street, followed by his melt down through drink and drugs excesses were funny in the movie. If you read his books though, you get a deeper insight. His recent efforts to clean up his act after prison have resulted in him developing a Sales Training Course called the "Straight Line Persuasion". There's great stuff in there.

I probably relate a little to Jordon Belfort, although my mad times were mainly prior to my business career. I made an effort throughout my career to try and learn, grow and develop. Most of the self-development material out there is focussed on the mind and body.

In fact, all the preceding motivational material is great for day-to-day improvement, but I was very fortunate to have come across a book called The Grail Message "In the light of Truth" by Abd Ru Shin. I found this book through the bass guitarist in our band, Dave Ross, after we had split the band up. This book was a "tough love" read which at age 25 I definitely needed. Dave and I were very close. Dave died in 2015 after a stroke and I miss him a lot. We saw each other at our best and some of our worst drug addled states. The Grail Message is a work for the individual and very spiritual, but practical in nature. This amazing book has become part of my life, and at age 56, I am still regularly going back into its pages. Not religious but spiritual in nature, it rings every bell for me and has made me a better person (I hope.)

It is impossible to summarise The Grail Message in a few paragraphs, and even if this whole book was written about The Grail Message, I could not do justice to its contents. It's personal to each person who takes the time and effort to read through it. I have read it many times and it will always be a part of my life. Not a philosophy, but a stand-alone work which has helped me make some sense of much of today's present day confusion. I was attracted immediately when the author stated in the opening paragraph that he was not bringing a new religion and there should be no attempt by another human being to influence another, as we are all personally responsible for what we think, say and do. Good council with the extremism and lack of tolerance getting worse globally.

Mederi Theraputics USA

Another classic example of how important past relationships and delivery of results is can be found by the US company Mederi Therapeutics. This company is led by Will Rutan who was the Vice President of Sales and Marketing at United States Surgical Corporation when I was with its European arm - Auto Suture. Contacts again!

Will Rutan has a classic medical device background and was a real player in the success and sale of USSC to Tyco (Covidien – now Medtronic as per the first Ideas in Medicine story). After USSC, Will worked for Leon Hirsch, Bob Knarr and Turi Josefsen as an entrepreneur in residence at their venture capital group, JHK Investments.

Will's role led to several successful exits from investments. Among these successes were the sales of CryoGen (sold to AMS) and AngioLink (sold to **Medtronic**). Prior to leading Mederi, Will also served as CEO of MiniLap, a laparoscopic device company, whose product line was licensed to Stryker Endo under Will's leadership.

Mederi is a fascinating company whose classic **Idea in Medicine** initially went commercially wrong. The idea was to deliver radio frequency to the Lower Oesophageal Sphincter in order to tighten the sphincter and help prevent gastric reflux. This is a disease which impacts on life way beyond uncomfortable heart burn, but can lead ultimately to Barrett's disease and potentially Oesophageal cancer.

The product is called STRETTA. The company which initially brought this to market was called Curon Medical, and they ended up in bankruptcy in 2006. I suppose it could be said that there are no good ways to go out of business, but there are definitely bad ways to go out! Curon went out of business in the worst possible way. One day they were trading and accepting money from customers and the next day…. gone……nobody answering phones, emails etc. A real mess. The thing is that this was not due to clinical lack of efficacy - but most definitely their business model and expenditure versus sales was a disaster.

They had raised over $100,000,000 of investment funds and managed to plough through that with extravagant ease. Then Will Rutan was brought in by a clever group of investors to resurrect the technology. Will was initially interested in the second product called SECCA for Faecal Incontinence but was convinced by a French Professor and worldwide expert in Gastric Reflux, Jean Paul Galmish from Nantes, that he should absolutely re-launch STRETTA as well. Professor Galmish noted exceptional results in clinical studies he had conducted and drew Will's attention to the need for a treatment like STRETTA.

What was initially thought to be a rather small re-launch project of Stretta, required significant capital and a virtual "do-over", with back to the drawing board efforts to redesign the products. Among Curon's mistakes was their sales model of offering free capital equipment in return for purchase of the disposable components. This "razor/razor blade" model has been utilized successfully many times. However, in Curon's case, the free capital was very expensive, and the company had negative gross margins on the disposables. The more they increased sales, the quicker they ran out of money! Mederi at great expense, redesigned all products for significant positive margins and did away with the free capital policy.

Mederi also segmented the Gastric Reflux market to focus on applications without competition. These were in-patients who had previous Gastric Reflux surgery called a Fundoplication. This is where part of the stomach is wrapped around the lower oesophagus. These were not candidates for revisional surgery. Also, people who have had weight loss surgery and had large portions of their stomach removed, rendering other methods of treatment impossible—except for STRETTA. The joint effect of a good business model and wise market segmentation allowed Mederi to capture the interest of surgeons worldwide.

Will's use of industry contacts (including yours truly) helped Mederi launch in 50 countries through distributors who often had a USSC background, and through surgeon relationships was able to get Medical Society backing for clinical use of Mederi products. Check out the Dr Oz PR recently on the www.mederi-inc.com web site. That was independent of any Mederi input!

I am part of the Mederi project and have been for 4 years now, helping by doing what I do: Distribution Management, clinical support and sales. It is always a great pleasure working with somebody like Will who has the same training and high expectations of delivery of results. Now, another name from the past, Bob Knarr is the CEO as Will has become the Chairman of the company.

What is nice about my business relationships is that many of them, over time, turn into true lasting friendships. It is certainly the case with Will and myself. He recently attended my daughter's wedding in Scotland with his childhood sweetheart Bonnie, and I was invited to a remembrance memorial service for his recently deceased parents in Blue Hill Maine. Our families all know each other and I am sure we will stay friends for the rest of our lives.

Kardus Medical, Turkey

Another dynamic businessman I met some years ago is based in Istanbul. His name is Bogac Ozdamir. In the sector of medical distribution there are many companies I could mention and many business owners. These relations tend to come and go depending on the projects underway.

Bogac started working in Ankara as a pacemaker specialist with Sorin Medical and one of the key people for ensuring import rules were followed. Sorin were briefly part of J&J and then became independent again. He had to place the orders and then ensure compliance to make sure that the import went smoothly and goods were not retained in Customs. Bogac was always ambitious and has a really sharp mind. As well as holding down a full-time position in Ankara, he started studying for an MBA.

Like I used to do with US Surgical, he was attending pacemaker implantations (in competition to the mighty Medtronic) and follow up controls for patients. He travelled to many cities in Turkey while doing that. In 1998, he left the company for 8 months for his military service and picked up his business again in 1999.

Bogac did very well and was soon asked to move to

Istanbul to work as an Area Manager. It was a very big decision for him to move away from home, but also a good opportunity. He was hesitant at the beginning and didn't want to settle down in Istanbul. His boss told him "if you want have a quiet, easy life and work as a line manager, stay in Ankara; if not, then you have to go to Istanbul".

So, a bit like my early days moving from Aberdeen to Glasgow, Bogac moved from Ankara to Istanbul. Also like me, he stayed in a cheap hotel for almost 3-4 months. He moved between both main cities and then made the move permanent to Istanbul. All the time I have worked with Bogac, he has been based in Istanbul.

For 10 years following that stage of his career he worked for Reysas-Data Medical as an area manager. His main business was Cardiac Surgery and mainly working with Datascope. Then in 2009, Bogac started his own company after being offered the exclusive distribution rights for Marmara region which bridges Asia and Europe. In fact, it's the most densely populated areas of Turkey. Bogac and I started working on the Surgical Sealant provided by Tenaxis Medical which was right in his target spot product wise.

In 2014, he was awarded the exclusive rights for Sorin Biomedical. When you deliver results, your name is never far away from the big projects. His latest achievements are introduction of the Endoscopic Vein Harvesting and Extracorporeal Membrane Oxygenation systems to Turkish Hospitals. For the last 2-3 years, he is focusing on Minimal Invasive Surgery with the continuing training to doctors.

Then came work for a global company called Emergo. He was helping a friend initially and didn't ask for payment. Then he was offered to be the main representative for Emergo in the Country and Region.

He is doing extremely well with Emergo and this impressive company provides service options for many of the tasks I need. Emergo work in most main markets globally in the Medical Device Industry, and they assist with device registration, quality compliance, in-country representation, regulatory advice and processes, distribution assistance and also can provide re-imbursement advice. This type of work is essential, as even in the EU, individual countries have their own registration and re-imbursement needs and can vastly differ from neighbouring countries.

In Turkey, there is now a national database covering all individual medical devices. Registering is mandatory, and there is little chance of building sales of a product there unless you get this element right. On the other side

112

Bogac, is helping Turkish manufacturers to get the necessary Free Sales Certificates, registration of their products in many countries and helping during the CE/FDA processes. All essential for export.

I could go on and name many other distributor companies like Bogac's, but this book would be like War and Peace. One company worth a mention is Lamed in Germany. The company was founded by Lazaros Ayvatoglou in Munich Germany. Lazaros started in medical devices many years ago and in fact helped establish Gore Medical and their range of grafts. His company has established itself as one of the best in the sector. I am sure he won't mind me mentioning his General Manager Ingrid Frank. Ingrid is extremely talented and one of the reasons for the well-managed company Lazaros owns. When you have met Lazaros, you will never forget this larger-than-life character.

Another company I currently work closely with is Healthware India Pty. Formed as a partnership between Ram Narayan and Shankar Rao they have built a sizeable operation with clients such as Olympus, Dornier, EMS and Mederi to name but a few. They are true professionals and have helped me understand the complexities of the dynamic Indian market over the last 12 years.

Ram's son Tarun is now working in the business and the

company has a real family feel albeit they employ around 200 people.

Ram and Shankar also enjoy a nice single malt whiskey and we have enjoyed a few drams over the years.

I have worked in 55 countries in the last 5 years and know specialist distribution companies in every one. So, if you are not mentioned please forgive me. You will be in the next edition!

Pluromed, LeGoo and Sanofi Biosurgery

Paris, France - March 16, 2012 - Sanofi and Pluromed Inc. announced that they entered into a definitive agreement under which Sanofi is to acquire Pluromed Inc., a medical device company based in Woburn, Massachusetts. The acquisition was subject to customary closing conditions.

Pluromed had developed a proprietary polymer technology, called Rapid Transition Polymers (RTPTM), pioneering the use of injectable plugs to improve the safety, efficacy and economics of medical interventions. Sanofi decided to buy the company and commercialize Pluromed's oddly named LeGoo®, a highly innovative FDA approved and CE marked gel for temporary endovascular occlusion of blood vessels during surgical procedures. Here is part of the news release;

"The acquisition of Pluromed underscores Sanofi's commitment to strengthen its Biosurgery portfolio," said Alison Lawton, Senior Vice President and General Manager, Sanofi Biosurgery. "LeGoo® is a breakthrough technology with the potential to change the paradigm of vascular and cardiovascular surgical procedures, by providing fast, temporary control of blood flow while avoiding vessel trauma associated with standard of care." "The synergies between our companies were clear from the beginning," said Jean-Marie Vogel, Chief Executive Officer of Pluromed, Inc. "We are confident that Sanofi has the expertise and resources necessary to bring LeGoo® to market and drive adoption."

"LeGoo® represents a major advancement in surgical technology because of its ability to control bleeding without clamps or snares that can injure delicate blood vessels," said Dr. William E. Cohn, Director, Minimally Invasive Surgical Technology at the Texas Heart Institute in Houston and a member of Pluromed's Board of Directors. "This breakthrough gives surgeons a way to temporarily stop blood flow into the surgical field which is imperative for clear visualization and accurate placement of sutures. I believe this technology will be widely adopted in cardiovascular surgery and perhaps in other fields in the future."

This acquisition reflected Sanofi's commitment to bring innovative solutions designed to ease surgical procedures and improve patient outcomes. I was very excited when this acquisition took place. I had met with the inventor and entrepreneur John Marie Vogel when I was working with LMA Urology as I advised the board of LMA to buy Pluromed. At that time, they did not have LeGoo but a product named "Backstop" which was designed to stop the migration of kidney stones in the ureter when lithotripsy was used to break the stones up. I remember we did some lab work in Miami as part of our due diligence. Boston Scientific currently sell and market Backstop. A missed opportunity for sure.

Jean Marie and his great VP of business development John Merhige went on to develop and name LeGoo – because the product is "gooey" and John Marie was French – hence "LeGoo"

Weird and catchy name, but LeGoo® is an amazing cutting edge technology. It is a thermo-sensitive biocompatible and non-toxic liquid gel that forms a plug when injected into a blood vessel to temporarily stop blood flow. It's an amazing **Ideas in Medicine** project and creation. The plug dissolves rapidly via cooling or spontaneously after several minutes. Once dissolved, the plug cannot reform because the concentration is too low. In a prospective, randomized study, LeGoo® was shown to provide better operating conditions than conventional occlusion techniques, by limiting blood flow into a surgical field without causing damage to the vessels. The study also showed a reduction in the time required to perform an anastomosis for beating heart surgery when using LeGoo®. Time is critical to patient outcomes in these types of surgical interventions.

Sanofi, a global and diversified healthcare leader, discovers, develops and distributes therapeutic solutions focused on patients' needs. Sanofi has core strengths in the field of healthcare with seven growth platforms: diabetes solutions, human vaccines, innovative drugs, consumer healthcare, emerging markets, animal health and the new Genzyme. Sanofi are investing in their future by looking for all the latest **Ideas in Medicine** that fit their global strategy. I met an amazing Executive there called Rachel Sha, a very dynamic professional who will go very far in the medical device industry if she chooses to, based in the hub of many medical start-ups: Boston – where Harvard University sits and Cambridge is chock full of innovative start-ups.

The really sad thing about the Pluromed/Le Goo story is that one year after successfully selling his company for a reputed $150 million to Sanofi, Jean Marie drowned in a boating accident. What a tragedy. He was such a character and had been around me for nearly 14 years in some capacity or other. As I mentioned at one point, I was encouraging LMA to buy his company. Talk about a lesson in enjoying the moment and living each day to the full.

Bionova Australia

Another project I was brought in to help with came along at the time of my departure from Tenaxis Medical. I had been a full-time Sales and Marketing Director with Tenaxis Medical, as previously mentioned, and Bionova was a perfect project for me. I was also retained by Sanofi Biosurgery to help manage their distributor base on a part-time basis. In fact, I ended up being the last Pluromed person retained by Sanofi for about two years after the acquisition. I loved my experience with Sanofi.

Bionova was an Australian, Melbourne based company, which was small, under-resourced and short on capital. It had survived for many years on a shoestring, but the idea was brilliant. This **Ideas in Medicine** development was started by a cardiac surgeon in Melbourne Australia. He started the project to try and develop vessels for cardiac bypass procedures, but never quite got there due to the smaller lumen vessel required. He did however successfully develop a graft for peripheral bypass procedures and then Arterial Venous (AV) Fistula grafts.

I was brought in as per usual to help them with Sales and Distributor management. They couldn't afford to pay me full-time so we agreed a part-time retainer and healthy commission. I also did my best to try and find them a

120

buyer/investor who could bring this fine product to a better place in terms of global use. I had got to know George Le Maitre and Dave Roberts (Acquisitions and Mergers of Lemaitre) through my time at Tenaxis. I had set up a German Distribution deal with them.

Anyway, in Prague during a break at the European Endo Vascular Society meeting, I spent some time with Dave. It was clear he was interested in Bionova and I am sure LeMaitre had the company on their radar for some time. We chatted about the product which everybody knew was excellent. Dave was clearly knowledgeable about Omniflow. Any company worth its salt knows what is happening in their space and market. Lemaitre are a rapidly growing company and have enough resource to research market opportunities and potential. In 2014, the following press announcement was made.

"In an attempt to expand its portfolio of peripheral vascular devices, Massachusetts-based **LeMaitre Vascular, Inc.** acquired Xenotis – better known globally as Bionova, the manufacturer and distributor of the Omniflow II vascular graft – for $7.7 million on Aug 14, 2014. Per the terms of the transaction, LeMaitre made an upfront payment of $5.1 million to Xenotis. Moreover, LeMaitre assumed $1.2 million of Xenotis' bank debt and is scheduled to pay an additional $1.4 million by Aug 13,

2015. Xenotis (Bionova) is an Australian company with 10 full-time employees. It produces the Omniflow II biological graft at its facility in North Melbourne, Victoria.

For the fiscal year ended Jun 30, 2014, Xenotis (Bionova) generated $2.3 million in revenues compared to $64.5 million clocked by LeMaitre in its most recent fiscal year ended Dec 31, 2013. Xenotis (Bionova) sold 95% of its products through distributors in fiscal 2014 and currently enjoys regulatory approvals in Europe, Australia, New Zealand, Canada, Brazil and several other overseas markets.

Per the LeMaitre management, "Xenotis's Omniflow II vascular graft used for peripheral bypass and dialysis access is a natural match for LeMaitre's XenoSure biologic vascular patch used for precision endarterectomy and vascular reconstruction. The fact that Omniflow II has already been implanted 20,000 times since 1990 further vouches for its popularity among physicians and makes it a prized catch for LeMaitre."

As I had too many other commitments, I had already resigned my commitment with Bionova the year before in 2013. I was pleased for the shareholders, although some of the employees, most notably the sales and marketing Director, Craig Newton, was left a little high and dry. Craig had not been happy for some time but his hand was forced and he had to go along with all the other employees. Le Maitre had their own people and as is often the case they wanted to do things differently. I am in touch with Craig regularly and am putting a few projects his way. Craig is another professional it was, and is, a pleasure to work with.

Le Maitre certainly acquired a great product, and as we speak, the Aussie dollar has plummeted in value, making the export of goods more attractive for foreign market end user prices for the OmniFlow 2 graft.

And so the story of the surgical staplers moves on. USSC was bought by Tyco, changed its branding to Covidien and now Covidien has been acquired by Medtronic

Medtronic USA and Ireland

As previously described, Medtronic Plc. is (now) an Irish company with its principal executive office in Ireland and operational headquarters in suburban Minneapolis, Minnesota and is the world's third largest medical device company. In 2015, at the time of its acquisition of Covidien, Medtronic's market cap was about $100 billion while the market cap for CRH, Ireland's largest indigenous business, was $18.4 billion. Medtronic operates in more than 140 countries. The company employs over 85,000 people and has more than 53,000 patents.

Talk about **Ideas in Medicine**! As previously mentioned, Medtronic was founded in 1949 in a garage in northeast Minneapolis by Earl Bakken and his brother-in-law Palmer Hermundslie as a medical equipment repair shop. They originally wanted to sell basketball pumps due to a shortage in the Midwest in the 20th century. Bakken began as a graduate student in electrical engineering at the University of Minnesota before he gave up his studies to focus on Medtronic.

The company expanded through the 1950s, mostly selling equipment built by other companies, but also developing some custom devices. It built a headquarters in the Minneapolis suburb of St. Anthony in 1960 and moved to Fridley in the 1970s. Medtronic's main competitors in the cardiac rhythm field include Boston Scientific and St. Jude Medical. In 1998, Medtronic acquired Physio-Control for $538 million. The company remains focused on the mission originally written by co-founder Bakken in the early 1960s The first sentence of the six-paragraph mission statement reads:

> *"To contribute to human welfare by application of biomedical engineering in the research, design, manufacture, and sale of instruments or appliances that alleviate pain, restore health, and extend life."*

After the 2008 global financial crisis, Medtronic stock value dropped dramatically. Despite sales and margins being well above the average of most industries, with steady revenue growth and a gross margin generally above 60%, Medtronic initiated a series of restructurings in 2008, 2009, 2010, and 2011, including Physio-Control's spin-off for $487 million and the stock price now approaches pre-recession values.

I am detailing all this so you can see how a small idea realised can become a monster success, although many changes, acquisitions, restructuring etc. are often essential to ensure ongoing growth.

In May 2014, Medtronic agreed to pay over $1 billion to settle patent litigation with Edwards Lifesciences after years of protracted legal battles.

Then, In June 2014, Medtronic announced its acquisition of Covidien, PLC of Ireland for $42.9 billion in cash and stock. Following the acquisition, Medtronic ceased to be a Minnesota-based company, officially renamed Medtronic PLC and headquartered in low-tax Ireland.

So now, Medtronic owns USSC/Auto Suture, having been bought by Tyco, then converted to Covidien after a branding change. And USSC/Auto Suture started with an idea and the creation of a now globally accepted surgical technique called surgical stapling. An initial idea, plenty of hard work, creative minds, overcoming challenges and billions of dollars have been changing hands. Real business creating real jobs and massive clinical and patient benefit.

So think back, my entry into the medical world with USSC/Auto Suture has been previously detailed. Along the way, numerous lasting and firm relationships and friendships have been maintained. Today, the initial **Idea in Medicine** created in a garage to develop the first practical heart pacemaker has grown into an entity big enough to have spent billions to acquire my original company. Medtronic is now one of the largest medical device companies in the world.

HoverTech International

Another client I have helped over the years - and am still active with - was developed by an Engineer and Entrepreneur, Dave Davis. As patients around the world become heavier and bigger, the need to move them safely has become essential. His **Idea in Medicine** which he brought to an amazingly successful level addresses the important issue of patient transfers.

In the late 1970s, the owner of an old flour mill with a paddle wheel and wooden floors was attempting to unload a boxcar full of specialty flour. For some reason, the pallets of flour were on top of a floor of inflated tire inner tubes. While attempting to get the small electric pallet truck under the inner tubes, one inner tube popped and scooted across the floor like a rock skipping over the water. The idea was born that using the controlled force of the release of air from a piece of fabric would make moving heavy loads easier.

Campbell Soups heard of this technology and hired an independent engineer to investigate its usefulness in moving pallets around the warehouse. Sometime later, the engineer's father-in-law was admitted to the hospital. While there, his daughter was asked to leave the room so the nurses could transfer her father from bed to stretcher. She stayed and saw a very difficult, uncomfortable transfer. She came home so distraught that she said to Dave "Why don't you do something useful with that air thing you're investigating?"

Hence, David T. Davis, Future President and Founder of HoverTech International, started his career in air-assisted lateral transfer devices. After quite a few years, Dave decided to launch the HoverTech International family of products, with the introduction of the HoverMatt. Because he believed in helping people, Dave knew he could make improvements in both the lives of the patient and the care-givers. So, he took the risk and started Hovertech International (HTI).

Working around the clock to sell and manufacture his product, it was slow at first, but Dave knew he had the best product and he could help so many caregivers and patients to avoid injuries. There was an overwhelming need for this product and Dave had the overwhelming desire to meet that need and help as many people as possible. Like so many of the innovations and **Ideas in Medicine** in this book, the path to acceptance is long and arduous. Effectively, the market has to be created. However, when the concept is clearly of benefit, slowly but surely, the Idea becomes a gold standard, and it's almost as though the product has always been there.

So, as time passed, HoverMatt caught on and Dave was able to move the business from the little house they started in to a bigger house. Still working around the clock, he continued to connect with as many caregivers as possible to teach them how the HoverMatt could change their lives and protect them from back injuries.

Dave also sold other non-HoverMatt products to nursing homes to help fund the start-up and expansion. To save money, Dave sometimes slept in campgrounds instead of hotels. HTI was totally self-funded by saving money from commission checks from the other products he was selling.

Dave bought a used sewing machine and taught his step-daughter how to make the HoverMatts. Dave would make the air supplies at night. When sales increased, Dave taught a sewing factory how to make the product and had someone else make the air supplies. Now, HTI has a factory in California, one in Taiwan and three factories in China making the HoverMatts and a factory in Taiwan making the air supplies.

Dave slowly began expanding the representation of the product through people he met at various trade shows.

This is where I came in. I was helping an ex colleague Charles Reynolds build his UK Distribution company in

Scotland. Charles has always said I gave him his first start when I promoted and recruited him for the Vascular Therapies team in USSC Auto Suture.

Charles asked if I could help his sales in Scotland where he already had customers but needed more of a focus. I sold the Hovermatt and especially the single-use versions to every major NHS Trust in Scotland. This was very satisfying, and I have since moved on to focussing on International Sales expansion for HTI.

HoverTech had three employees and about 15 independent sales reps at their first sales meeting in 2011. Now, HTI has 24 employees and 70 independent sales reps in the US with international sales in Australia, UK, Kuwait UAE, Saudi Arabia, France, Germany, Spain and other countries. The HoverMatt is recognized as the number one choice of hospitals for lateral patient transfers, boosting, turning in bed, positioning in the OR. The product line has increased to include the HoverSling, the HoverJack, the HoverMatt Half-Matt, and the HoverMatt Split Leg. Many of these products are available in both reusable and single-patient use versions. The Evacuation HoverJack is used by Emergency Medical Services. Dave is always looking for ways to improve current products along with adding new ones to preserve

HoverTech's reputation as the leader in air assisted lateral transfer devices.

I have had great pleasure in participating in the global growth. I have just closed a deal for Medpharma in Barcelona where Falcke, the huge Danish Ambulance company has bought three systems for their ambulances specifically prepared for obese patients.

So, from an idea to commercialization, Dave has created a multi-million-dollar trading company. He recently turned down an offer of close to $100 million for his company as he is so passionate about what he does and its positive impact on patients and health professionals alike.

I am editing this section in San Antonio prior to Hovertech's largest ever event in March 2016

A perfect **Ideas in Medicine** story.

More valuable than gold.

One of the amazing things about the medical device industry - and it's becoming even more apparent as I write this book – is how important friendships and contacts are. If you deliver results and don't let people down, then your reputation is enhanced. Unpopular people are quickly isolated from the players. I am very lucky that I have a core of top quality contacts that are feeding the growth of my business. I service their business growth needs and they reward me in return.

Whilst at Arab Heath in 2014, I was introduced to Guðmundur Fertram Sigurjónsson (Fertram) and Ivar Thor Axxelson (what a great name) – two fine gentlemen from Iceland Fertram had founded a company called Kerecis. Dr Eyad's (storyline coming) team had monitored their progress through the FDA (US Federal Drug and Administration authority) notifications and Dr Eyad wanted the Kerecis product range for the Middle East.

Ramsay McLellan, mentioned earlier, was also at the Arab health congress, developing markets for his Ideal Omega fish oil range. I asked Ramsay to sit in on the meeting with the Icelandic delegation. As well as the skin graft, they had four unique CE marked dermatological creams. Ramsay became very excited about the creams. The

133

creams are unique as Kerecis have a patented process of including fish oil in their creams (high in Omega 3) without any fishy smell. Kerecis have gone to the expense and trouble of CE marking each individual cream for the specific ailment it helps. The creams are effectively class 1 medical devices instead of being a cosmetic cream. They treat eczema, psoriasis, calloused feet and ingrowing hair – all major global skin problems.

Following the meeting, it was clear Ramsay could assist with the roll out of the cream project because of his vast array of contacts in the Omega 3 world. Ramsay has since developed some global initiative to ensure sales internationally become widespread.

Iceland catches a lot of cod, an average of almost 300,000 tonnes of it per year in fact. There is a huge waste associated with that. Enter Guðmundur Fertram Sigurjónsson and his team of scientists who devised an ingenious use for all that previously wasted fish skin.

If you remove all the cells from fish skin — the unused residue from fish processing — you are left with a simple cell-free structure that is rich in Omega 3 fatty acids.

Apply this biologic bandage to a wound, and it will incorporate into the body in a natural way, the fatty acids nourishing and enhancing a speedier recovery.

This is the idea behind Kerecis, a 20-person company on the cusp of greatness. With a patent for using intact de-cellularised fish skin as a treatment alternative for people with severe tissue damage, and some small but encouraging clinical trials behind them, the group led by Fertram is about to expand into new markets. My son Christopher is now part of the Kerecis team. Over a few beers in Munich around April 2014, I was discussing my 18-year-old and his prospects in the UK. Fertram said "why don't you send him up to Iceland as we desperately need people".

The next day, with a bit of a hangover, the conversation was the first thing I thought about, but I was not sure that it was just the beer talking. Anyway, Fertram immediately said "send me Christopher's CV". Within two weeks, Christopher had been interviewed and was offered his first full-time job living in Isafjordur way up in the North West Coast of Iceland. Christopher is loving his job and life in the small village of Isafjordur where the Kerecis plant is based. Pure seas, pure living and good people. Fertram always said "if he can survive an Icelandic winter, he will do well". We are Scottish and used to hard winters, but often Christopher had to dig himself out of his house to get to work and dig the snow away again to get home! So, Kerecis is getting a lot of my attention right now as I am so grateful for the personal opportunity they have given my son.

The market driver behind the concept is the growing diabetes epidemic (for example, up to 20% of the population of the US could have developed the disease in a few short years). Many diabetics suffer from chronic wounds, and some of them must face amputations if traditional wound care approaches are unsuccessful.

The Kerecis' strips of sterile fish skin are inserted into these chronic wounds. The product attracts healthy cells almost like a skin graft. The clinical trials to date indicate that the products might be more efficacious than the closest biologic alternatives made from pig products.

Its source is one of the appeals: fish skin does not have the religious barriers associated with pig products, and it has a secret ingredient, Omega 3 fatty acids, that also help to treat inflammation in the wound. Furthermore, there are no viruses that can travel between fish and humans making the product saver to use than pig sourced alternatives.

In addition to its efficiency, its production is sustainable. After all, this is a product derived from something — fish skin — that otherwise goes to waste in the general fish processing process. But, Fertram says proudly, "one gram of a Kerecis wound strip is worth more than gold".

With his strategic recruitment of my son, Fertram has ensured he gets the skill and effort of a full-time Sales and Marketing Director to help his company grow. It is a terrific Ideas in Medicine idea, and I am plying my trade to help them expand in many markets. Fertram quickly realised how I could help them and made me a share offer which gives me real long term reasons to help the company grow and succeed.

With FDA and European approval, and sales already established in Iceland, Europe and the Middle East, Kerecis is now ready to expand its offering.

"Our mission really is to document cases where we have prevented amputation," says Fertram in a recent interview. "Then you can see the product in use. There are people who are miserable and afraid of losing their limbs and then you see them use our product, and that's a really wonderful feeling."

A great company where the original **Ideas in Medicine** has led to global patents and expanding product lines. The American Military have just invested a seven figure sum in Kerecis to research the effect of Kerecis Wound in trauma and burns.

Things are changing rapidly, and in October 2015, my old boss – and now one of my closest friends – Lars Mikkelsen was in Reykjavik for discussions with Kerecis. Let me tell you about Lars.

Lars became my boss in Auto Suture. There were some management changes when I was a rep with the company. It was a tad acrimonious, and during the changeover when my original General Manager Sue Titterington was "let go", we had an end of year dinner for the whole company at the Turnberry Hotel in Scotland. ALL the men were measured and dressed in Kilts regardless of their nationality.

Lars was advised by me how to dress like a true Scotsman. During the evening as the drink flowed, he kind of forgot, and some of the female marketing team got more than they bargained for as far as his Norwegian manhood was concerned. He was sitting slouched back with his legs wide open! Traumatic for the girls!

Anyway, I was at the top table next to Turi Josephson one of the Auto Suture (USSC) – now Medtronic – come on keep up! founders and owners. Lars was across from me and Sue was at the table. Out of blue Lars said "Graeme, please stand up and make a speech thanking Sue for all she has done for the company". To say I was surprised – and of course totally unprepared – is an understatement.

I stood up in front of a hundred or so company employees and made an impromptu unprepared speech. I think it went down well. There were a few teary eyes as Sue was well respected by the team.

The reason I was at the top table, was partly due to the fact I was again the top sales performer. I was up for a special award called the President's Award. I was very proud of what I achieved in Auto Suture. It was an extremely demanding, performance-oriented, environment. Fail to achieve your sales number a couple of quarters and you were usually let go. They did not tolerate lack of success.

Lars and I became close in 1996 thanks to our main competitor. The company Ethicon, part of the global medical giant Johnson & Johnson had noticed I was taking a lot of their business. They also noticed they could not take any of my business. I had always ensured my day-to-day activities went way beyond the normal dedication for duty. I worked hard at providing a top level clinical service. The Surgeons and Nurses looked at me as part of their team. I was scrubbed and assisting every week. The sales came because of that.

So, when Ethicon came with a "name your price" employment offer, I was flattered. Of course, I mentioned their approach to my line manager. Then when it got back to Lars, an interesting thing happened. Lars's secretary called me and said that Lars wanted me, Catherine, Emma and Christopher in Oslo – the whole family. I was to meet with Lars Monday. We flew Friday and he had us stopover in Copenhagen for a night. All expenses paid in business class for all four of us. I still remember Christopher who was only 2 years old sitting proudly in his own business class seat.

What was Lars doing? Lars was being very clever. The family had a ball and Catherine suddenly liked the "new regime" – she certainly hated the old one because families were irrelevant to the achievements demanded. The company had one of highest divorce rates in the industry. Lars and I met on Monday and he didn't even offer me an improvement in my package but he wanted to explain what he had planned for me if I continued to excel.

He knows now that I never had any intention of leaving Auto Suture for our only competitor. My credibility would have been shot to pieces with the clinical teams I had supported and trained for years with the Auto Suture equipment.

Lars, was great to work with and he and I built a true friendship and we always had great fun while getting our business done. Some of my worst ever hangovers have been following nights out with Lars. Norwegian and Scots drinking habits are similar – bad – but similar.

So now, Lars and I are back working together and we will help build business in Scandinavia for Kerecis. He has always loved my family and the fact that Christopher is working for the company gives him added incentive too.

Lars recently left a position as Vice President of Mediq a large €6 Billion turnover Dutch owned company and he has numerous projects underway including helping Venture Capital firms close deals and assisting the Norwegian Health Ministry with their efficiency drives. Lars is a true professional and will always do well.

We are already planning our next liver challenging get together somewhere in Scotland, Norway or elsewhere.

Dr Eyad Al Saleh and the Middle East

Dr Eyad Al Saleh found out about me and sent an employee of his to seek me out as he wanted a product I was working with.

The product was Pluromed's uniquely named Le Goo product as previously described. This was an **Idea in Medicine** of a truly unique nature. A quirky, brilliant extrovert French man called Jean Marie Vogel had developed this from his first **Ideas in Medicine** invention called Backstop. This was a product I had come across before and had encouraged LMA Urology to look at acquiring.

Backstop was designed to be injected in the ureter behind a urethral stone to stop it being pushed back into the kidney during Lithotripsy. It would have been perfect for our Stone breaker device. What a combination. At that time without any commercial sales or success, Jean Marie wanted $7-9 million for his company Pluromed. It was too steep for us and there were many unanswered questions about the gel being used and its effect on the body. I was with Udo Roslan, another ex-colleague of mine from USSC – who has since tragically died. He had a heart attack aged only 50 – what a shame. So many ex USSC people have surfaced in leading roles and I had worked with Udo in various roles in various projects.

Anyway, I remember saying to Jean Marie he was asking too much money. Little did I know he was developing LeGoo for Vascular and Cardiac use which caught the attention of Sanofi Bio Surgery and he subsequently sold his company Pluromed for a reputed $150 million. After Sanofi bought the company, I was retained by Sanofi to manage the Distribution network. I was surprised, as I was sure Sanofi – with 80,000 employees would have their own people to do what I do. I ended up being the last Pluromed worker to leave Sanofi. I enjoyed my time working with Sanofi which I did on an outsourced task-orientated basis (no time expectations of one or two days a week etc.). Most tragically, Jean Marie Died a year after becoming a multi-millionaire when he drowned on Lake Michigan where he was boating in his new boat. All the above previously mentioned but it is an amazing story

Dr Eyad wanted LeGoo and he sent his man to meet me. Daniel tracked me down and we eventually met in London. After discussions with Daniel, it was clear I should meet Dr Eyad who owns a very successful and lucrative medical business called AMG based in Kuwait. Dr Eyad also has operations throughout the Gulf Cooperation Council (Saudi Arabia, Kuwait, UAE, Qatar, Oman and Bahrain). Dr Eyad is also the Chairman of a major

Canadian mining PLC.

During the annual event in Dubai called Arab Health, Dr Eyad usually takes a suite at the 7 star Burj Al Arab Hotel. He arranged to meet me in his two-storey private suite. In full Arab robes, he cut a fine figure and massively impressed me with his vision and ambition to "make history"!

Dr Eyad as well as being a highly successful business man is a Professor of Gynaecology and Clinical Oncology.

Dr Eyad has since become a very important part of my own business and life. I always enjoy being with him and his amazing capacity for big vision "big brush" expansion plans. He is motivational to be around, and his keen intellect coupled with a deep spirituality are a great balance for any human being.

I am a part of those "making history" plans, and I am proud to have brought some very high revenue producing lines to his Portfolio including Mederi, Alesi-Surgical, Bio nova, Clear flow, Celsius Medical, Hovertech, Combat Medical, Kerecis and Norman. As a medical doctor, he quickly spots the winning lines and his ability to penetrate his markets is legendary.

Normon pharmaceuticals in Madrid is one of our key

projects. He is taking their lines into Kuwait. The Normon facility is 80,000m2 of some of the most modern generic pharmaceutical manufacturing in Europe. The new factory was opened by the Queen of Spain in 2013. The factory is owned by the family Govantes and Victor's (connection coming up) Uncle is the CEO. A family company in the true traditions of the name.

Medpharma and Spain

Dr Eyad asked me to be the CEO and sole Director of a Barcelona-based company called Medpharma. Dr Eyad invested in this company to build a business servicing Spanish, European and countries further afield. Medpharma is a work in progress, but you can be sure we will make this a success as Dr Eyad has "making history" aspirations for this part of his operation too.

The Spanish connection is great for me as I love the country and we have a villa in Andalucia which we designed and built about 15 years ago. I have many friends also in Madrid and our lawyer is based in Madrid. Arturo Fernandez is a tremendous asset and is now a friend. As well as having his own practice, he lectures in Civil and Commercial Law to the Law students at Madrid University.

The main hub around many of these Spanish connections – in fact Arturo was introduced to me by this friend of mine – is Victor Govantes. Victor is part of a classy Madrid family. I know his Dad, also Victor Govantes, his Mum Maria and sister Diana Govantes. Victor is a dynamo. Later in the book you will hear how one of his projects is now a very important one of mine.

Victor's global contacts are legendary, including royalty in Saudi Arabia, Dubai, Abu Dhabi and the "royalty" in Madrid. As well as the actual royal family, there is hierarchy in the city which is akin to the UK "connections club". Victor's family are involved in some of the largest businesses in Spain including pharmaceuticals, laboratories, manufacturing and retail chemist shops.

British Innovation

Another example of how important it is to maintain friendships and relationships in this industry is a British **Idea in Medicine** Ultravision. David Frederick (yes, the one with the weak constitution) is currently the Chairman and brought in by the Venture Capital company IP Group. His vast experience was seen as essential to the success of this venture. David then called me and said come and meet the CEO Dominic Griffiths and help us expand our International Distributor network. This is classic from Eureka to Commercialisation **Ideas in Medicine** launch.

Both Dominic and David are great to work with, even though they can be demanding at times. In fact, my wife Catherine calls Dominic my "work wife" as he is on the phone so often.

Ultravision is the invention of Dr Neil Warren, Head of the Welsh Institute of Minimal Access Therapy (WIMAT), Cardiff University. It is a revolutionary product for handling the surgical smoke that is created during laparoscopic surgery, a modern technique for performing minimally invasive surgery in the abdominal cavity.

Smoke produced by modern "electrosurgical" instruments during laparoscopic surgery rapidly builds up and severely impairs the quality of the operative visual field. This makes surgery inefficient and unnecessarily risky to the patient.

Furthermore, although many workplaces have adopted smoke-free environments, surgical staff continue to be exposed to surgical smoke. This is unpleasant for the surgical team and chronic exposure may have long-term health implications.

Ultravision rapidly and efficiently clears the smoke as it is created whilst simultaneously preventing its release into the operating theatre. This innovative new system therefore addresses a universal and significant problem in the seven million laparoscopic surgery procedures performed annually, and whose adoption will benefit patients, surgeons and nurses.

Initially working with funding from the University's own seed fund, an initial prototype was developed in 2009 which yielded promising results in experimental models. A subsequent equity investment funding round by two investors – IP Group and Finance Wales – resulted in the formation of the spinout company Alesi Surgical Limited in 2010.

Development of Ultravision continued within Alesi Surgical. The company collaborated with the University throughout development. This has involved both expert consultancy and a range of experimental work. All of this work was critical in ensuring that the product is both safe and meets the needs of the surgical team. The continued relationships with the University via Dr Warren of the Welsh Institute of Minimal Access Therapy(WIMAT), the technology transfer team together with essential interactions with NHS surgeons in Cardiff has led to the development of the product and its subsequent approval for launch in January 2014.

Ultravision is the first product to be launched by Alesi Surgical. It has helped to raise the profile of surgical innovation at Cardiff University, of WIMAT as a leading surgical training centre, and the medical device sector in Wales as evidenced by the following:

- Winner, 2013 Royal College of Surgeon's Cutlers prize for 'best surgical invention' (March 2014).
- Winner, Praxis Unico Business Impact (Aspiring) Award 2014

Since approval of the CE mark in January 2014, the penetration of the market has required a fundamental change in the business as it transitions from a largely "virtual" entity to one that can support a rate of growth.

The company now has a team of eight employees and is seeking to recruit additional resources to help drive future growth. I have helped Alesi Surgical identify and appoint 19 distributors covering over 25 countries worldwide.

The successful development of Ultravision enabled the Company to raise £6m in equity investment from its investors IP Group and Finance Wales. The vast majority of these funds have been spent within Wales and the UK.

The company has already been discussing an offer of £20,000,000 for their technology from a Tier One Company and our goal is to build it, increase its value and see how it values in 2 or 3 years' time.

Annual Global Events

Every year, there are a number of "must attend" congresses which I go to. Most of my clients have specific congresses orientated to the surgical specialty they serve. This is where they meet the doctors who will use their technology. The biggest Congress/Exhibition geared toward country distributors is Medica and it's held every year in Dusseldorf Germany. It's always in November and it's usually cold, always dark, usually raining and often snowing! This Congress is so huge that there are up to 28 Congress halls filled with Manufacturers from all over the world. Every major manufacturing country has its own Pavilion. So the USA, UK, China, Russia, Japan, Brazil, India etc.

Every Distributor looking for new product lines to sell will attend Medica to find and negotiate with companies looking to sell their lines! MEDICA attracts a great number of international experts. More than half of the approximately 130, 000 trade visitors came from over 120 countries. Also, the top decision-makers tend to be at Medica. Over 5,000 global manufacturers will present their new products and services to highly qualified clients from all across the world. Lectures and presentations take place directly in the exhibition halls, offering an exciting addition to the trade fair happenings. From medical technology to research and healthcare industry start-ups right up to physiotherapy. MEDICA remains a top platform for all the participants of the world market for medical technology and medical products.

There are other trade fairs such as Arab Health in Dubai every January and Hospithera in San Paul Brazil every May. Then there are all the surgical speciality congresses such as Digestive Disease Week which attracts up to 22,000 doctors and is in a different US City. In 2015, it was in Washington DC where I am writing this paragraph.

In fact, there are 1,000 different medical congresses all over the world every year. An industry within an industry. Companies pay thousands and thousands of $$$ to sponsor these events, pay for staff hotel rooms, entertain staff and medical professionals. It is truly amazing how so many of the valuable medical congresses just would not take place without industry sponsorship. So many surgical and medical innovations would not see the light of day without this sometimes incestuous and essential relationship.

Looking back, I have attended these events for over 20 years. Many of the senior decision makers started off just like me in a sales role. They have walked the walk and know I have done so too. I have lost track how many, dinners, lunches, breakfast, coffees etc. have been enjoyed to help create deals.

Travel Diary....... "Whickers World" with Proper Work Not Just Sightseeing.

When looking back on the countries I have had the privilege of working in – some of them on numerous occasions – the memories fade as to how tough international travel has become. I have travelled on numerous occasions in First Class and Business Class with airlines such as Emirates, BA, Qatar, Cathay, Virgin, Singapore, Thai, Iceland Air, KLM, Air France and Turkish.

Make no mistake, I have also travelled in economy and budget airlines such as Ryanair, Easyjet, Germanwings, Air Berlin etc. It's the one element of my planning that is difficult to delegate to an assistant. Unless they have travelled extensively, the "tricks of the travel trade" are hard to ask anyone else to organise. As well as the flights, another essential element are the hotels. My favourite chain is Intercontinental, but I have top tier frequent stay cards with the Hilton and Marriot groups also.

I have literally earned millions of air miles and hotel points. My family, over the years, have loved helping me spend on them with trips to China, Vietnam, Thailand, Mexico and numerous visits to different parts of the USA and Europe being at least part paid for by the travel I have enjoyed – or often endured!

It's not easy anymore (was it ever?), but the security checks and queues are tough regardless of the class of travel. Priority lanes and airline lounges definitely help, but it still hard going.

A recent trip to Erbil in Kurdish Iraq highlighted the growing security issues. I was only 40 miles from Mosul which is still controlled by the ISIS extremists. I was well protected and always felt secure, but the airport security was something else. Two vehicle checks before arrival at a security building over a mile from the terminal but also within the fenced off airport grounds. Two further checks there after which we travelled by an airport bus to the terminal where a further two checks took place. I predict this is likely to be duplicated in other high-risk airports as our world becomes more chaotic.

Friends and colleagues often comment on the glamorous locations I travel to and the beautiful hotels and restaurants I stay and eat in. Not many would jump on a plane to Kurdish Iraq right now though and so I have to "pay the price" for international business when demanded. However, to me, it's all necessary to maintain my international pedigree which is a large part of why companies want to contract with me.

The one thing that's become a bit of a joke and self-fulfilling prophecy is that I am a hopeless queue chooser.

If you are ever behind me in an airport or hotel check in and you see me choosing a passport control or security check queue, then do yourself a favour and go in a different line. The line I am in inevitably will move the slowest or have an "issue". Don't remind me of the power of thought forms as I have tried everything! It must be karma or something!

I am writing this on the way to Abu Dhabi and flapping a bit as I look at my diary. I have trips pending to Barcelona, Dusseldorf, Munich, Warsaw, Izmir, Erbil, Madrid, New York and Hyderabad. My Indian passport has run out and now the Indian government gives me two-year multiple entry visas. It helps, however, it's still a logistical hassle. Both my passports are nearly full again and I will need one for my planned travel while the other is away for the Indian Visa. The UK Government has allowed me to carry two legitimate UK passports because of these situations. Many people don't realise you can have two passports and it certainly isn't common, but if you write to the Passport office with supporting evidence of past and pending travel they can make exceptions. I have had two passports for around 10 years now.

What's Going On Now?

Ideas in Medicine are manifesting everywhere. Dr Eyad's research team have discovered a new client called Admetsys a Boston-based start-up.

The Inspiration behind the company began with a frustrated intensive care nurse's challenge to an endocrinologist:

"I have a diabetic being treated with intravenous insulin. His glucose levels are up, down, and all over the chart. Once an hour, I have to leave another patient to measure his glucose, then read two pages of complicated orders— just to change the insulin rate. If you doctors are so smart, and with all the technology out there, why isn't there a machine that will control glucoses for me?"

That nurse's frustration was well justified. In the last three decades, the diabetic population has exploded; however, the methods and tools for diabetic control in the hospital have remained essentially unchanged. The current standard of care is highly labour-intensive, requiring manual blood sampling, glucose measurement, dosage calculation, and treatment adjustment by a nurse—optimally once per hour.

Reliance on this chain of tedious manual processes limits precision, permits errors, and risks dangerously low glucose levels from overtreatment. Moreover, lack of measurement automation means remote monitoring and alerts simply do not exist for inpatient diabetic care. These circumstances represent a crucial, unfilled gap in the standard of care with unacceptably high costs.

The technology is protected by two patents, one for the system itself, and one for the proprietarily differentiated consumable supplies. Patents on all the core technology have been approved in both Europe and the United States. Moreover, patent protection is not the only safeguard: all consumable supplies are designed with encrypted electronic chips that uniquely identify them to the system, eliminating medication delivery errors and preventing any attempt to use supplies not certified by the manufacturer.

On the Finances & Investment, Admetsys is raising a $500k convertible debt round to accelerate its production engineering and support its European clinical trials planned for launch in November at Kolding Hospital.

A subsequent Series A money raise of $7 million will be required to achieve market clearance both in the Europe and the United States, with commercial launch in select European markets. These objectives would position the company strongly to raise future growth capital, as well as make the company highly attractive to potential acquirers.

The management team is led by Jeff Valk, Chief Executive Officer, a seasoned leader of highly technical organizations, and a hardware and software engineer specializing in design of adaptive systems.

Research and clinical operations are headed by Dr. Tim Valk, Chief Scientist, a board certified endocrinologist, researcher, and former professor with over 25 years in clinical practice.

Regulatory, supply chain, and internal operations are headed by Glenn Robertelli, Chief Operating Officer, a medical industry veteran and global supply chain expert.

The work is starting with this exciting new **Ideas in Medicine** company. I am looking to help them raise money and expand their sales base though appointing distributors. Also, to help establish some local clinical trials.

The thing is, it's all about friends and contacts again. Dr Eyad's research team found Admetsys. In Kuwait they have one of the highest – if not THE highest – diabetes rates in the world with about 1 in every 2 adults in the Kingdom a diabetic. This is truly an explosion of epidemic proportions. The Admetsys **Ideas in Medicine** can help clinicians in the country cope better, help patients and control costs.

Who knows where this innovation will lead? But one thing's for sure – I hope to be involved.

Spectrascience Inc, USA

The latest **Ideas in Medicine** project is one close to my heart after my own cancer incident.

SpectraScience, Inc. was formed from the combination of assets from GV Medical, a Minneapolis-based company and MediSpectra, which operated in Boston, MA.

Both of these failed start-up companies were using light technologies and the interaction of that light with human tissue to discern information about the tissue. MediSpectra had developed a light-based system to screen for cervical cancer. The initial thought was to replace traditional colposcopy with their system. GV Medical was independently developing a different light-based technology in order to diagnose small polyps and lesions found during colorectal cancer screening.

In 2005, the combination of these two entities was re-launched as SpectraScience, Inc. and located in San Diego, California. The focus of the newly formed company was to commercialize light-based technologies for use in the detection and diagnosis of a variety of epithelial cancers. That remains the mission of the company today.

At United European Gastroenterology Week (UEGW) 2012 the company introduced the WavSTAT4^R Optical Biopsy System and I was introduced to the CEO and President Michael Oliver in Barcelona at the 2015 United European Gastroenterology Week. I was introduced to Michael by another ex-Auto Suture colleague Hughes Wielemans. The old contact network working again. As the product is CE marked, SpectraScience are able to sell in many parts of the world including the Middle East.

The product uses a technology known as Laser-Induced Fluorescence Spectroscopy to directly measure the concentrations of certain bio-markers in epithelial tissue. The first indication of use is for the diagnosis of small and diminutive polyps encountered during colonoscopies conducted in the course of normal screening for colorectal cancer.

 An optical fibre, contained within biopsy forceps, is introduced through the working channel of the scope into the colon. The optical fibre is placed in contact with the polyp to be diagnosed. A footswitch is activated, pulsing laser light from the console's light source, through the length of the fibre into the polyp.

The pulsing laser light excites certain amino acids and enzymes found in the tissue. As the bio-markers absorb energy from the light, the electrons in the outer shell of

163

these compounds moves to a higher energy state. When the light is turned off, the excited electrons, return to their original and normal energy states.

In making this transition, the electrons emit photons of energy. Those photons are captured by the optical fibre and transmitted to a spectrophotometer contained within the console. Analysis of the fluorescent signature by a very sophisticated mathematical algorithm results in a digital value that can be used to make a very accurate determination regarding whether or not that specific polyp has characteristics that make it possibly pre-adenomatous or whether it is simply hyperplastic. That determination is made in approximately 1 second.

Clinical studies with literally thousands of specimens have shown a Negative Predictive Value of the WavSTAT system from 93-98%. The threshold for clinical acceptance as determined by the American Society for Gastrointestinal Endoscopy (ASGE) is a NPV of 90% or greater. ASGE also recognizes that moving to non-invasive optical biopsies is faster for the clinician (1 second response time), safer for the patient in that unnecessary biopsies and the resultant complications are avoided, and less costly for the health care payers. This again is a classic **Ideas in Medicine** concept in action.

The company also has white light technologies that utilize Scattering Spectroscopy to measure nuclear sizes of cells to determine their likelihood of being pre-cancerous as well. Scattering spectroscopy is particularly suited to conditions such as determining whether or not dysplastic tissue is present in a particular sample. The application for this variant of light-based technologies is in the diagnosis of dysplastic tissue in Barrett's oesophagus, a pre-cursor of oesophageal cancer.

This particular indication would replace the random biopsies of the oesophagus that is associated with screening of Barrett's patients today. Those costly, painful and time-consuming biopsies are repeated at regular intervals as the patient undergoes surveillance for this condition. While not all patients with Barrett's Oesophagus progress to oesophageal cancer, those that do can make the transition to cancer in situ very quickly. Oesophageal cancer is one of the fastest growing diagnoses in oncology today. It is also a cancer with a very low 5-year survival rate.

Recent studies conducted by renowned urologists have determined that light-based technologies can also discriminate very accurately between malignant and non-malignant lesions in the bladder. In order to make an accurate diagnosis today, a fluorescent dye is injected into the patient.

After several hours, the dye will concentrate in the bladder, illuminating any lesions that may be present. The uptake in malignant lesions is different from benign lesions, allowing the clinician to differentiate between the two when viewed through a cystoscope. Using the natural fluorescent nature of the tissues without need for artificial fluorescent enhancement allows the procedure to be done without the introduction of expensive drugs. Drugs that can often cause harmful side effects.

SpectraScience is on a mission to deliver information to the clinician regarding the detection and diagnosis of suspected areas of cancer. Their goal is to make these determinations accurately, cost-effectively, and in real time to provide clinicians worldwide with the information they need to treat their patients. With faster, less expensive and safer diagnostic modalities, we can find cancer earlier, treat it sooner, minimize trauma to the patient and, most importantly, allow more patients to survive their encounter with cancer.

This is a project I am very happy to be working on and I will use my experience, contacts and International reach to help SpectraScience establish a good business platform.

As usual, the goal is to find suitable and appropriate distributors for each country SpectraScience asks me to develop.

Seeing the Light

Back in the Medicapro days in 2003-2006, we were building the GX Labs biocide range and I had approached a company called Vernon-Carus early on who were interested in our products.

This privately owned healthcare business (sales to 50 countries) were a great platform for our non-alcohol based range. Bruce Ash the CEO had recruited a new Executive Director and board member called David Ford. David took over the management of the project and his intelligent "can do" attitude transformed our progress.

Vernon-Carus was successfully sold to Synergy Healthcare Plc in November 2007, attracting a premium value.

David called me during the end stages of writing this book. He is involved in four main medical device projects at Executive and board level. A couple of these projects he founded himself. David is another classic example of Ideas in Medicine in motion! He called to see if I would be interested in helping a new UK start up called Active Needle Technology.

After leaving Vernon Carus, David joined the British Standards Institute as an Executive Director.

The British Standards Institution, an independent organization established more than 100 years ago, has tremendous experience in the creation and implementation of all types of standards, both in the UK and globally: they operate in more than 100 countries. Engagement with BSI gives their customers the differentiating 'edge' to succeed in highly competitive environments.

David was responsible for all of the BSI Healthcare and Testing Services business worldwide. Medical devices and healthcare are an important sector for the BSI Group.

The capabilities of the British Standards Institution are amongst the most highly rated in the world. They grant companies the licence to trade in some markets and give them a competitive advantage in others.

In 2009, David formed a specialist global healthcare division in the BSI Group business, emphasising the position of BSI as a world-class certification and accreditation body to the Healthcare industry.

The work by BSI's two Notified Bodies (supporting the European Medical Devices Directive and the FDA) ensured that the world's leading medical companies had effective and rapid market access to key markets and health systems, get products reviewed with technical competence, integrity and independence. David also worked for – guess who – the mighty Medtronic between 1999 and 2003 and ran their Cardiac Division.

Anyway, David called me to discuss a spin off from a company called Lightpoint Medical – Active Needle Technology. David is a board member for Lightpoint Medical. As mentioned earlier in the book, SpectraScience are also using light to detect cancer. The coincidence and timings are interesting. This is a non-competing company.

Lightpoint Medical is an innovative medical device company dedicated to improving health outcomes for cancer patients through image-guided surgery. The Company's proprietary technology, based on Cerenkov Luminescence Imaging (CLI), has the potential to help guide cancer surgery, providing more accurate treatment whilst sparing healthy tissue.

Differentiating cancerous and healthy tissue intra-operatively can be an issue. At Lightpoint Medical, the aim is to bring light to this surgical challenge through the use of molecular imaging in the operating room.

The company was founded in 2012 to develop products with the capability of detecting cancer in real-time during surgery. CLI enables optical detection of Positron Emission Tomography (PET) imaging agents, with the potential to combine the simplicity of optical imaging with the high diagnostic performance of PET imaging.

Again, because of my own experience with the big C, this project gets my attention.

Surgery is a commonly used tool for the treatment of certain cancers. Unfortunately, the goal of removing all cancerous tissue is not always achieved, and either the surgery has to be repeated or the patient's subsequent treatment pathway is amended. Confirmation that any excised tumour has a margin of healthy tissue is the key criterion for surgical success.

Although there are techniques and equipment available that provide some information regarding margin status during the procedure, none are considered reliable, practical and easy to use during surgery. Today, surgeons primarily rely on visual and tactile assessment to find cancerous deposits.

The LightPath™ Imaging System is designed to fill this important medical need. By providing a means to assess tumour status intra-operatively, via molecular imaging, it aims to enable surgeons to know with confidence that they have removed all cancerous tissue.

The system detects Cerenkov Luminescence, a faint light produced by PET imaging agents widely used in cancer diagnosis. Although the science behind the LightPath™ system has been known for many years, this is the first time that it has been utilized in this way and the LightPath™ Imaging System is the first approved medical device for intra-operative molecular imaging in the world. The technology provides the potential for optical imaging of numerous cancer types.

So, David Ford introduced me to the CEO of Lightpoint Medical David Tuch. David T. is a Harvard Medical School and MIT graduate and scientist. He came from positions in Novartis and GE Healthcare and has a deep understanding of imaging and physics.

Active Needle Technology www.activeneedle.com is a spin off from Lightpoint Medical www.lightpointmedical.com .

Active Needle Technology (ANT) is an innovative, early-stage medical device technology that has a proprietary medical device platform technology for the accurate imaging and placement of needles during patient biopsies and which represents a significant improvement over currently available technologies.

It has a broad application, but in order to maximise success, the initial product offerings will be in cancer biopsy.

The technology addresses a pressing medical need for better tools to detect cancer in the early diagnosis phase, a phase upon which all further treatment options depend.

Active Needle Technology exploits conventional Doppler ultrasound technology: by imparting ultra-frequency pulsation to the needle itself. This limited, but highly rapid, longitudinal movement of the needle renders an otherwise invisible needle clearly detectable.

The company is currently focused on developing the technology in the field of cancer biopsy, not only because of the growing medical need and potential for high downstream sales, but also because of the near term, non-diluting funding opportunities available in the field of cancer research.

This spin off for LightPoint Medical will be driven by the CEO Ian Quirk. Ian was a Director of LightPoint Medical and has been asked to lead the project.

Ian has experience in a variety of medical device start-ups in such areas as coronary, peripheral vascular, active implantable devices, in vitro diagnostics, orthopaedics and spine and interventional radiology.

The team has considerable expertise in obtaining funding and support for medical device start-ups.
Other opportunities, which may be pursued once the initial offering is commercialised are in the fields of anaesthesiology and maternal-fetal medicine.

The technology has achieved pre-clinical (cadaveric) proof-of-concept using a prototype device developed for anaesthesiology and as of February 2016, in core needle biopsy.

Active Needle was developed in Dundee University by Dr Muhammad Sadiq.

David T. and Ian have asked me to join the board of this exciting start up in order to offer guidance in terms of route to market and commercialistion. They are a great group of professional medical device executives.

Again, it's all about contacts and relationships. Thanks to David Ford for the introductions and reference. I will do what I do and focus on what I am good at – building business platforms for sales.

This part of the book is being written during a break in a lecture for a clinical training in Izmir, Turkey on a Saturday morning. The course is a joint course between Mederi and MMS (a Dutch diagnostic company) and has 18 visiting doctors. Even here, a doctor spoke to me about an idea she wanted to develop. It's happening all the time.

We are about to treat patients with the STRETTA device and Professor Bor always likes me in the treatment room to ensure the equipment is functioning well for the patient.

My clinical support is still an important part of my client support activity.

Recently, as our accountant Kate Baxter said when she saw some pictures of me in a Hospital Support environment in the OR. "There was me thinking all you did was travel the world flogging stuff".

The "flogging stuff" is part of it for sure, but as the business is developing, there are many more angles.

I am personally investing now in businesses. Some quite diversified and not strictly in the medical device arena but consumer-orientated.

Victor and the Govantes family, as mentioned earlier, have created a business called DeLabCare srl. Its web site is www.delabcare.com. One of the key lines is a series of soothing balms for the rapidly expanding tattoo industry. The product is called Balm Tattoo, and in addition to providing creams to soothe the skin after a tattoo, it will also help to prevent infection. The business has exploded in Spain and we have already established companies in the UK and USA.

We want to create a cleanliness standard and envisage a "kite mark" standard on a tattoo parlours door. This would indicate that as well as having great tattoo aftercare products for the skin, the parlour would have protocols to ensure clean hands, clean instruments and clean floors and surfaces. We have been talking to Paul Blenkinsopp (remember the MedicaPro story) who is Sales and Marketing Director for Ebiox www.ebiox.co.uk . They have a unique range of non-alcohol products and a unique biocide. In addition to having this unique range, we will provide a range of alcohol-based products for the more cost-conscious parlours. Also, a quality line which is being distributed by Covidien (now Medtronic) in Spain.

Ramsay who you heard about earlier has a new business venture called Clever Shave www.clevershave.com. Basically, it's a business giving people an opportunity to have a great shave every day, save money on their razor blades – men and women – and help the environment at the same time. I am helping us adopt some unique angles and the medical device experience is helping as we are looking to provide cleaning and sterilising fluids as a consumer product. My experience with Tim Rogers in GX Labs will help us find the right product, price plan and product benefits for a full range of soaps, pre shave and after shave products.

After the course in Izmir, I travelled from there to Medica Dusseldorf for the biggest annual medical device exhibition in the world. I met many of the people mentioned in this book, and who knows how many new projects will unfold. Certainly, many of the existing ones will be progressed.

Events are moving on and ever changing. On a personal note, I am now officially a proud Grandfather to Erin Rose MacNeil. My daughter Emma gave birth in the hospital you read about earlier – the Southern General Hospital. After massive development and investment, it is now the Queen Elizabeth University Hospital Glasgow. A fine facility. That hospital was the first place I saw general surgery performed, was the place David Frederik and I met, and now my fabulous daughter Emma has given birth there. She did so well. Max, her husband, was by her side the whole time. My wife and I spent 7 hours there in maternity waiting for Erin to make her arrival into the world. As we walked around the new facility, many of the Victorian buildings I had spent hours of my life in are being knocked down and replaced with state-of-the-art facilities. We walked around on a sunny and chilly Sunday morning nervously waiting.

That's also the place where I went when my testicular cancer was first checked out by the surgeon Kuram Mir.

That very same facility where the team allowed an examination is boarded up and about to be bulldozed.

I have spent hours and hours of my life in hospitals, and to be around this hospital again for such an exciting reason was strange.

It was all slightly surreal.

My courageous son Christopher has left Iceland and is now engaged to Georgia, a lass he met in the village of Isafjordur. He moved to England and was offered one of the first jobs he applied for. He told me recently that the fact he had the strength of character to move to Iceland and work there stood him out from the numerous other applicants.

I have been formally offered and accepted the board position with Active Needle Technology. A number of the people you have read about in this book gave references which the CEO said were "glowing". Nice! This represents a new chapter in my business life. One which Markus Haller said about a year ago is the natural progression for somebody like me. I had a great call with the newly appointed Chairman Mike Hawley. He's a South African who has lived in the UK for many years and has broad and extensive medical device experience. His vision for the project is exciting. I am looking forward to learning from this talented group. To always be learning is another lifestyle attribute which is healthy to maintain.

As I said, my business life is an ever-changing landscape. The ability to accept change is one thing I have always felt comfortable with and is a good attribute to attain to.

The business platform of **Ideas in Medicine** is there for you if you have your own Eureka moment and need to find a trustworthy source to help develop your idea. We won't be able to develop every idea, and there are many other people out there who can help. However, at the very least we might be able to point you in the right direction

I hope this book has shown how my own experience in the dynamic medical device industry may be able to give you confidence that at the very least, you can explore your own idea. You may have the next success story. You won't know until you try.

Ideas in Medicine are occurring every minute of every day somewhere in the world.

I hope to be part of yours.

Contact us directly through; www.ideasinmedicine.com

Or our Twitter account; @ideasinmedicine